Philosophical Dimensions of Personal Construct Psycho

T0256257

Since its formulation by George Kelly in the mid-1950s Personal Construct Psychology has been distinguished by its links with general philosophy and by the philosophical richness of its fundamental postulates. Personal Construct Psychology recognises that any attempt to understand why we behave as we do must begin with an understanding of how we create meaning. After a brief general introduction Bill Warren traces the philosophical history of Personal Construct Psychology through the broad and complex tradition of phenomenology and thinkers such as Spinoza, Hegel and Heidegger. He also gives credit to the influence of general creative and dramatic literature across a variety of cultures. Specific issues addressed in depth include the position of Personal Construct Psychology with regard to philosophy of science, cognitive science, clinical psychology, concepts of mental illness and the implications for social and political philosophy.

Philosophical Dimensions of Personal Construct Psychology will provide counsellors, therapists and students of Personal Construct Psychology with a broader appreciation of its historical and philosophical context and its importance to contemporary psychology.

Bill Warren is Associate Professor in Education at the University of Newcastle, Australia.

Routledge Progress in Psychology

Emerging Patterns of Literacy
A multidisciplinary perspective
Rhian Jones

Foundational Analysis
Presuppositions in experimental psychology
Pertti Saariluoma

Modelling the Stress-Strain Relationship in Work Settings
Meni Koslowsky

Philosophical Dimensions of Personal Construct Psychology
Bill Warren

Family Argument
Dispute and the organization of domestic identities
Charles Antaki, Ava Horowitz and Peter Muntigl

Philosophical Dimensions of Personal Construct Psychology

Bill Warren

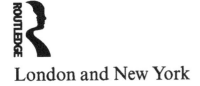

London and New York

First published 1998
by Routledge
2 Park Square, Milton Park, Abingdon, Oxfordshire OX14 4RN

Simultaneously published in the USA and Canada
by Routledge
711 Third Avenue, New York, NY 10017

First issued in paperback 2014

Routledge is an imprint of the Taylor and Francis Group, an informa company

© 1998 William G. Warren

Typeset in Times by Routledge

British Library Cataloguing in Publication Data
A catalogue record for this book is available from the British Library

Library of Congress Cataloguing in Publication Data
Warren, Bill 1942–
    Philosophical dimensions of personal construct psychology /
    Bill Warren.
    1. Personal construct theory – Philosophy. I. Title.
    BF698.9.P47W37   1998   98–17308
    150.19'8–dc21   CIP

ISBN 13: 978-0-415-16850-2 (hbk)
ISBN 13: 978-1-138-00712-3 (pbk)

[The suspension] of the 'subject' and 'self-understanding' . . . cannot mean that we should liquidate the subject (the actually existing industrial societies and the institutions of the 'administered world' are far more adept at this; why compete with them on the level of theory?); rather it can only mean that one has to explain subjectivity better and in a more adequate way . . .

(Frank, 1989: 343–4)

One cannot understand a spoken statement without knowing both its most general and its most personal and particular value.

(Schleiermacher, 1977: 48)

What is not supposed to be my concern. First and foremost, the Good Cause, then God's cause, the cause of mankind, of truth, of freedom, of humanity, of justice; further, the cause of my people, my prince, my fatherland; finally, even the cause of Mind, and a thousand other causes. Only *my* cause is never to be my concern. 'Shame on the egoist who thinks only of himself!'

(Stirner, 1845: 3)

Contents

Preface   ix
Acknowledgements   x
A note on citations   xi

Introduction   1

1 Locating philosophy   8
History   8
Developments   11
Domains   16
Modes   19
Concluding comment   21

2 Links and latencies   23
Direct references   23
Latencies   29
Constructive alternativism as philosophy   48
Realism and idealism   52
Concluding comment   60

3 Constructivisms   61
Social theory   61
Psychology   65
Concluding comment   72

4 Structuralism and beyond   73
Structuralism and poststructuralism   75
Modernity and postmodernity   78
Psychology and postmodernity   80
Concluding comment   85

5 The problem of the self   **87**
   The notion of the self   87
   Decentred and recentred subjects   92
   Constructing selves   93
   The self in personal construct psychology   99
   Concluding comment   103

6 Philosophical psychology   **105**
   Philosophy of science   105
   Cognitive science   109
   Determinism and free will   116
   Philosophical issues in clinical psychology   118
   A caveat   120
   Concluding comment   126

7 Psychotechnology   **128**
   Psychotechnology, applied psychology, technology   128
   Personal construct psychology and applied psychology   131
   Personal construct psychotherapy as praxis   *135*
   Concluding comment   139

8 Political and social life   **141**
   The social-political in personal construct psychology   141
   The egalitarian outlook   145
   Ideology   146
   Religion   150
   Concluding comment   154

9 Being human, making meaning   **156**
   Hermeneutics   158
   Personal construct psychology and hermeneutics   164
   Psychological philosophical anthropology   166
   Concluding comment   169

Conclusion   **171**

References   174
Index   192

Preface

I came to personal construct psychology from a background jointly in social philosophy and a fairly traditional 'psychology is a science' education in psychology. I had been led to existentialism and to anarchist thinking by my preoccupation with the subtleties of individual interpretation in and of life. Personal construct psychology was discovered, by accident, during my education and training in clinical psychology. It appeared to offer a congenial way of thinking about individual lived-experience in a most thoroughgoing way. It appeared also to be consistent with the types of ideas generated in the anarcho-psychological tradition of western thought with which I had become familiar. Thus developed an interest in probing personal construct psychology for its links to the ideas generated in this tradition and in social philosophy generally.

There is now something of homelessness felt by those with an outlook that is fascinated by individual variation, recalcitrance, endurance, resistance, and the like. The intellectual climate is one in which the dominant wisdom accepts a more collective view of human beings; thus, it would take those with such an outlook to be naive and suffering from ideology. Still, there is something in lived-experience that resists the insistence on giving up the sense of difference and individual efficacy, of uniqueness and ultimate aloneness.

Thus, the present volume is an outcome of excavating the philosophical in personal construct psychology, and a construction of it in terms of a construct system the core constructs of which keenly focus *the personal*. A different construction, both of personal construct psychology and of life, would, obviously, understand matters differently; but the tolerance of difference and of plurality, might be the mark of an optimally functioning person and of a good approach in philosophy.

Acknowledgements

The preparation of this manuscript was made easier by a period of leave from the University of Newcastle, and I am most appreciative of the opportunities that leave afforded me. The work of others writing on themes to which this work is addressed provided much of the 'data' for the present discussion, and that work is acknowledged for the encouragement it provided. My thanks go also to Mark Ralph at Routledge and to the copy-editor, Justin Dyer, whose attention to the technicalities of the actual production of the work was greatly appreciated. Finally, I thank my family for their tolerance, and for their support during the completion of the project, which burdened them as much as it did me at times.

A note on citations

There are now two different editions of Kelly's original two-volume work, the 1955 W.W. Norton and Company edition, and the 1991 Routledge edition. Where these volumes are referenced in the text, page numbers in each are cited for convenience of those who have only one set of these volumes. Where two dates are cited for a source, the first refers to the date of original publication and the second to the date of the edition used. This second date is the one under which the source is listed in the Bibliography.

Introduction

George Kelly, in formulating the work that introduced personal construct psychology to the psychological community, felt more disposed to get on with the job of propounding his theory than paying respect to the pioneers of the approach he was to take. Thus has the theory of personal constructs been noted to have paid scant regard to the work of others. The present volume is intended as a contribution to filling this gap. Some four decades on, it is also of interest to consider developments since the original formulation and how personal construct psychology might respond to the challenges to thinking emerging in the period immediately following publication and reaching their full impact only after Kelly's death.

Since its appearance in the mid-1950s, personal construct psychology has attracted attention not only for its stated focus and range of convenience – psychology, clinical psychology and personality – but for Kelly's (1955/1991) preparedness to address the philosophical basis, and the philosophical location, of personal construct psychology. This was a bold move at a time when the rift between psychology and philosophy might have been seen as widening. However, in the event, it was a move that provided personal construct psychology with the soundest footing and a most congenial situatedness within a philosophical tradition that is particularly helpful for illuminating the human condition, both individual and collective.

This work is, then, in the first instance, in the nature of a philosophical compendium. However, as such a collection of observations and discussions of links and connections in respect of personal construct psychology and philosophy, it displays the philosophical richness of personal construct psychology. Thus, there is an argument in 'form'; that is, the range of matters in respect of which personal construct psychology has something to say supports a claim that personal construct is a psychology with significant philosophical respectability. It hopefully also shows its philosophical respectability at a time when philosophy and psychology as disciplines have become antagonistic, and a need for a *rapprochement* might be suggested.

There are also included here smaller arguments, perhaps sometimes 'suggestions', that proved too difficult to ignore or too attractive not to pursue. One concerns the clash between personal construct psychology and social constructionism. Here, it was impossible to resist addressing a *déjà vu* of older arguments between Marxism and theorists of the anarcho-psychological tradition; as well as to note philosophical difficulties within Marxism itself. Another concerns the idea of personal construct psychology as a clinical psychology, thought of as *praxis*. And there is a sketch of the development of hermeneutics to lend support to the view of personal construct psychology fitting most comfortably into the hermeneutic tradition.

Thus, the broader picture is that personal construct psychology falls in with a substantial tradition of thought about the human condition generally, and is broader and richer than its location as a 'mere' psychology might otherwise suggest. It contributes to a level of reflection on the fundamentals of the human condition that is, generally, the traditional domain of philosophy. In short, the significance of that move that Husserl discussed as a move from a concern with 'facts' to a concern with 'ideas' was that it threw humankind into a unique position that psychology has been ill able to illuminate. Personal construct psychology offers an illumination of the path this move put us on, an understanding of the individual which finds deeper questions and deeper understandings of their species 'immanent' within individuals' understanding of their predicament.

One risk in preparing such a volume as the present one is that it will not be comprehensive. This risk must remain that not every relevant contribution to the ongoing discussion of philosophy and personal construct psychology will have been considered. Where this is the case, the sin is one of omission not one of commission; that is, no judgement has been made about any such omitted contribution. Another risk in trying to draw so much material into focus is that the work might be found to raise connections, then leave them undeveloped. If the work does throw up ideas for others to develop, however, then well and good. Not only would such an observation be consistent with what is attempted here, but also it would be in the spirit of personal construct psychology itself. That is, personal construct psychology is a theory which encourages new ways of thinking about human psychological functioning and encourages experimentation with ideas and behaviour. Hopefully, the identification of relationships between personal construct psychology and different issues and perspectives in philosophy contributes to this ongoing process of elaboration.

These last comments recognise that the present work itself, as a discussion of philosophical issues in personal construct psychology, will be construed differently, and at different points, and by different readers. Thus, perhaps it might be overall understood as a philosophical 'conversation' with personal construct psychology and those who construe it.

The original intention of the volume was a focus on personal construct psychology, not on constructivism in general, nor constructivism in psychotherapy, nor on constructionism – if constructionism is seen as usefully differentiated from constructivism. It may well be that many of the connections drawn out here hold just as well for other forms of constructivism and for constructionism. However, Kelly self-consciously located his position in relation to philosophy, and his is arguably the only constructivist theory of personality *and* psychotherapy (Chiari and Nuzzo, 1996a), the only psychology for psychotherapy (Mair, 1970a), and one of few large-scale psychologies founded in human interaction (Butt, 1996). Thus, it is personal construct psychology with which we are here concerned, and an outline of how that concern is elaborated is as follows.

Chapter 1 is a quite straightforward account of philosophy in fairly conventional terms, reviewing its history, sketching its traditional concerns, and illustrating its modes of operation. This chapter could be omitted without loss by readers already even modestly read in philosophy.

Chapter 2 looks to specific observations about philosophy and personal construct psychology made from the outset by Kelly, and to latent dimensions teased out by others since the initial formulation. We do this in some cases in detail because often only a general acknowledgement or a brief account of a particular thinker is made by Kelly and by commentators on personal construct psychology. Here is also considered the possibility of locating personal construct psychology as a realist position. This is a controversial location and one that here draws on what is arguably the most thoroughgoing realist position in the work of the Scottish-Australian philosopher John Anderson (1893–1962). This might not clarify the existing debate, but it perhaps adds another interesting dimension to a discussion of it.

Chapters 3, 4 and 5 address matters that have been problematic in philosophy itself, and suggests how these might be dealt with in, or for, personal construct psychology. First, the social constructionist position is considered in terms of the social theory it appears to represent, partly at least, by reason of its own social-historical origins, and against the background of the realist position previously outlined in Chapter 2. Some of the different constructivisms in psychology are also noted for their fit with personal construct psychology. Second, the debate between a so-called modern and a postmodern way of understanding life is, bravely perhaps, considered in terms of some of its major themes and issues, and accounts of its significance for personal construct psychology reviewed. Third, growing directly out of these two chapters, in Chapter 5 a problematic notion is discussed that constructivism and postmodernity, but no less than modernity itself, have wrestled with; that is, the idea of the individual, the *self*, the Ego, or the subject.

Chapter 6 reviews some selected issues that attract the attention of those working in the field of philosophical psychology. The position of personal construct psychology in respect to philosophy of science, determinism and free will, and the most advanced thinking in cognitive science is surveyed. Further, given the focus of convenience of personal construct psychology, that is, clinical psychology, two matters raised by the philosophy of clinical psychology are noted: the concept of mental illness, and the problem of classification. We finally signal a warning; that is, a reminder of the problems philosophy has had with psychology since the separate discipline of psychology emerged and parted company with the discipline of philosophy. This reminder appears appropriate to avoid too grandiose a claim being made for personal construct psychology, particularly in view of its own focus and range of convenience being specifically limited to psychology.

Chapters 7 and 8 shift the focus to matters that have not been widely considered within personal construct psychology. First, the manner in which personal construct psychology avoids the critical thrust brought against many of the 'psychotechnologies'. This is linked to considerations in Chapter 6, but now an argument is added that personal construct psychotherapy is usefully thought of as a *praxis*. Chapter 8 examines what social-political implications might be discerned in personal construct psychology, or the implications it has for social and political philosophy.

In Chapter 9 a range of material is drawn together to provide an account of the development that was *hermeneutics*, and an identification of personal construct psychology in terms of this tradition. In turn, a suggestion is developed that personal construct psychology, understood in terms of this tradition, makes a contribution to a psychological philosophical anthropology. In this way, having been seen to have been sensitive to the three others of Kant's four fundamental questions of philosophy, it adds a perspective on the fourth; that is, the question of the *potential* of humankind.

While the first chapter acknowledges that some readers may not be widely read in philosophy, the work itself could easily fail to acknowledge that other readers will not be widely read in personal construct psychology. Thus, some effort should perhaps be made to provide a brief survey of what personal construct psychology is about. Numerous more comprehensive surveys already exist, such as Bannister, Fransella and Agnew (1971) and Dalton and Dunnett (1990), while other, more focused discussions provide outlines and overviews (for example, Part I of Button, 1985; Part I of Winter, 1992; Fransella, 1995). However, a brief sketch seems appropriate here.

Personal construct psychology fits into 'critical psychology' (Sullivan, 1984), a perspective that replaces organic and mechanical metaphors of the individual with the metaphor of the personal. This last metaphor stresses the significance of an irreducible I–thou dialogue that both defines the person and provides the social context of personal development.

In 1955, George Kelly (1905–1966) published the results of some thirty years' experience in psychology: a two-volume work titled *The Psychology of Personal Constructs*. The work is notably, and consciously, slight on discussion of other thinkers from whom he drew inspiration, a fact that prompts the present volume. Further, it has not been a significant part of the mainstream of psychology; more a tributary that has perhaps been dammed up. Neimeyer (1985) considered its 'sideline' status and suggested that it was significantly related to its idiographic emphasis. Further, he thought that it was 'too difficult'; it required a radical rethinking of what psychology was essentially about.

Personal construct psychology is more than a little difficult to 'type'. While

Kelly consistently and adamantly denied any connection with cognitive psychology, personal construct psychology is regularly claimed as a precursor of and an example of, the 'cognitive revolution' in psychology. Kelly (1955/1991) did, however, provide a thoroughgoing perspective for a rethinking of what psychology was about and how it was best done. This was stated as a fundamental postulate and eleven corollaries which can be summarised to provide an indication of the position with which we are here to deal in terms of its philosophical dimensions.

The fundamental postulate of personal construct theory is: *a person's processes are psychologically channelised by the ways in which he or she anticipates events.* This is a careful statement that succinctly captures a number of different things about our psychological functioning. Most significantly, it emphasises that the individual does not just *react* in terms of past experience but rather *evaluates* events or situations in terms of predictions about the future. The individual is seen as trying to make a sense of the world 'in advance', so to speak, of the next event or situation which will overtake him or her.

This postulate is elaborated through the corollaries which deal comprehensively with personal and, significantly as it turns out, interpersonal life. A *construction corollary* suggests that a person anticipates events by construing (placing an interpretation on) their replications, that is, the themes or recurrent events in the flow of experience. An *individual corollary* makes the perhaps obvious yet too easily overlooked point that persons differ from each other in their construction of events. An *organisational corollary* indicates that constructs are organised into different *systems* for different individuals and that these systems involve hierarchic relationships. Thus there is an idea of 'core' constructs which are more important to the individual, and of 'subordinate' constructs that are relatively less important. A *dichotomy corollary* stresses that a person's construction system is composed of a finite number of dichotomous constructs, that life is conceived in terms of *contrasts* between good and evil, ugly and beautiful, and so on. A *choice corollary* asserts that the alternative in a dichotomised construct is chosen in terms of the extent to which the individual anticipates the greater possibility for extension and clarification of his or her system. A *range corollary* emphasises that a construct is convenient for the anticipation of a finite range of events only. For example, 'respect versus contempt' may apply to a range of interpersonal relationships for one person, but be used only in relation to strangers by another. An *experience corollary* notes that a person's construction system varies as he or she successfully construes the replications of events. A *modulation corollary* stresses that variation in a construction system is limited by the flexibility or permeability of constructs, that is, the extent to which a construct will readily admit new elements to its range. The addition of a non-personal element like 'fire' to the 'respect versus contempt' construct above is an example. Thus, experience in a serious fire might see the construct widened in the sense of 'respecting fire' because, say, we now appreciate its potency. A *fragmentation corollary* clarifies how a person may successively employ a variety of constructive subsystems which appear logically incompatible. This stresses that change need not be 'logical', in the sense that different levels of construction may be involved across a series of events, uniting them in terms of an overarching construct; for example, the inconsistencies in parent–child behaviour of hugging, later smacking, later still ignoring, and then again manifesting concern (Bannister and Mair, 1968: 22). A *commonality corollary* concerns the level of social life. It notes that to the extent that a person employs a construction of experience which is similar to that employed by another, his or her psychological processes are similar to those of the other. Finally, the related *sociality corollary* states that to the extent that one person construes the construction processes of another, he or she may play a role in a social process involving the other person.

The model of the person in personal construct psychology is that of the person as 'scientist-psychologist', an active, meaning-giving, meaning-understanding creator who cannot be studied as an object (nor, for that matter, in terms of observed 'behaviour' alone). This model contrasts with the 'information processor' model of the person in the empiricist tradition. The meaning given to situations, events, and so on, is *individual* (though consistency across individuals occurs and provides the basis of social relations and role-playing), and is organised into a system (one of core and peripheral constructs) that will be more or less complex. In relation to any domain of experience and experiencing, a particular individual would be expected to have a more or less personal interpretation which was more or less complex. There may be 'core' constructs which the person could not change or could only change with great difficulty, peripheral constructs which would be more amenable to change, or a combination of core and peripheral.

Personal construct psychology is an attempt to deal with the whole complex of meaning-giving. What is given is an account of human behaving which comprehensively *encapsulates* the various aspects that psychologists and philosophers have tried to *isolate*: cognition, affect, volition. It is a disciplined study of the inner *outlook*, an alternative to the scientific psychologies of the outer inlook, and a *step beyond* the experiential psychologies of inner *inner* feelings (Kelly, 1963: 183). Moreover, in its therapeutic approach it takes significant account of a client's own inner outlook.

Personal construct psychology fits into that broad and complex tradition that is phenomenology, a tradition that can trace its concerns to Heraclitus, through Spinoza and Hegel, and which culminates in Husserl, Heidegger and the religious and non-religious existential phenomenologies. This is a rich if complex and confusing pedigree. Indeed, Kelly was concerned to place his perspective in the context of philosophical perspectives already developed, and to give credit to the general creative and dramatic literature of all cultures. All of this creative and dramatic literature was an attempt to make a sense of the human predicament, an attempt to which he saw personal construct psychology making a systematic contribution.

This, then, is a very brief sketch of the position the philosophical dimensions of which are in focus in this volume. Some further indications of its nature and range will emerge in the following discussion. However one evaluates that discussion or specific elements of it, the fact that such a discussion can be had at all in relation to a particular psychology, and was encouraged from the outset, is significant for claims about the philosophical integrity of personal construct psychology. Hopefully, what will emerge is a broader appreciation or a general 'feel' of the philosophical territory into which personal construct psychology takes us.

1 Locating philosophy

Any discussion that intends to focus on philosophical matters, and especially issues in contemporary philosophy, requires that philosophy be placed in its historical and conceptual context. This is either a mammoth task or a straightforward one, depending on the detail felt necessary. Here, we opt for a 'broad brush' approach to form a general, quite traditional overview for those whose primary orientation is more likely to be psychology than it is philosophy; together with a little more detail where matters are particularly pertinent to our wider concerns. The intention is to 'locate' our fuller discussion both historically and conceptually, as well as to advance the 'compendium' function of the present volume. This will provide some common ground so as to more fully develop the philosophical dimensions of personal construct psychology, as we draw links and connections to specific ideas, movements and personages.

History

Western philosophy is usually taken to have begun with the pre-Socratic Greeks whose questions arose from a concern to know the ultimate constitution of the *natural* world that confronted them. Only much later to be characterised as 'metaphysics', this quest generated theories of all things returning ultimately to one or other of the four basic elements of earth, fire, air or water, or theories akin, conceptually at least, to modern atomic theory. As Burnett (1914/1968) instructs us, Greek philosophy from Thales to Plato was dominated by one main question: What is real? Central to this question was the fact of change; everything with which the Greek thinkers were confronted did not stay the same and only Heraclitus appeared able to accept that one 'never steps into the same river twice'. The only thing that did not change was the principle of change, and so great a concern was this that Plato later argued for the existence of a world of changeless Forms as security against such a disturbing reality. He also wrote the *Republic* as an account of an ideal social arrangement whose basic structure did not change.

Yet, with the appearance of the great Socrates and through his debates with the Sophists in the fifth century BCE, the focus shifted to *human* concerns.

With the emergence of Athens as the dominant city-state in what is now Greece, scholars of various persuasions flocked to that city; in particular, some thirty or so thinkers who became the first professional teachers. Unfortunately, they took a name for themselves, Sophist, derived from the same root word as is 'philosophy', a word signifying 'wisdom'. Self-described 'wise men' had something of a disadvantage to overcome in the particular culture in which they found themselves, and varying degrees of competence and integrity amongst them aggravated this. Nonetheless, they often held their own with Socrates, and in the debates which come to us principally through the words of Plato, we see a new type of consideration attracting the minds of Greek thinkers: social and political concerns. Now became relevant questions of how social life should be organised, how power should be distributed in a particular form of social organisation, what conduct was justified in relation to one's interaction with others, whether that conduct approximated 'the good', how the young should be educated, how 'the beautiful' should be judged, what constituted justice, and so on.

The practical Romans spread the Greek learning, anchoring it firmly in *this-worldly* matters until Christianity emerged to become the official religion of the Empire, and creative western thought was stifled by *supernatural, other-worldly* concerns for over a thousand years. Initially, the older Romans had been complacent about the fascination of their young people for things Greek, but this complacency gave way to concerted efforts to prohibit or restrict Greek learning, to reverse the assessment of Horace that 'Captive Greece took captive her savage conqueror'. There appeared a 'home-grown' crop of scholars in the personages of such men as Cicero and Quintilian, but whatever the accomplishments of these men the eventual conversion of the Emperor Justinian to Christianity brought the Christian Centuries (Payne, 1967): thirteen hundred years of ambiguous and controversial impact on the development of western thought. Essentially, philosophers now worked within a tight circle of questions framed in theological terms, a context in which there was little to discover. All that was significant had been revealed and, in any case, it was not the real nor illusory reality of this world nor the thoughts of human beings about their social, political and psychological life that was important. What was important was to prepare for the next, 'truer' life by understanding God's wishes for how we should conduct ourselves in this life.

During this period, the dominant religious position of Roman Catholicism was challenged. Thus that view gave way to a view, after Martin Luther's reaction, that the Bible itself contained all one needed, and the role of a special mediator, a priest, was downgraded in Protestantism. Yet, Protestantism, too, was later to develop its own internal divisions, and, more interestingly perhaps, to find itself aligned with that social and economic development that was capitalism. In turn, capitalism's own views about the nature of humankind, about the individual, about progress, about our rights and power over nature, found Protestantism flexible enough to accommodate its imperatives. The title of Max Weber's great essay *The Protestant Ethic and the Spirit of Capitalism* (1904–5/1948) captures the modern link between religion and social life, a link which Marx was to elaborate somewhat differently. Interestingly, while Weber links two larger-scale *social* forces and concludes somewhat pessimistically for the future, Mitzman (1969) has drawn a direct link between Weber's social theory and his *psychological* state. Weber's personal and family struggles are argued to contribute to an attraction to a style of analysis and understanding of broader issues. This suggestion emphasises the interaction not only of mind and world in a general sense, but of a particular frame of mind and particular types of understanding and explanation. A similar though more general view is found in Popper's (1945) argument that those drawn to historicist views – that is, a belief in forces operating on our lives that we can little understand or influence – are attracted to a *methodological essentialism*, and to a *historicism*.

To return to our history, it was with Jean-Jacques Rousseau in the eighteenth century and a philosopher much inspired by him, G.W.F. Hegel in the late eighteenth and early nineteenth century, that *human* concerns reemerged as centrally important in philosophy. Equally, so did an interest in studying *this* world; an interest which gave a significant impetus to epistemology. Rousseau and Hegel are arguably the pivotal figures in the history of western thought in relation to educational thought and to more general philosophy, respectively. After Rousseau nothing would be quite the same in our thinking about education, which saw a major tradition develop out of his ideas; that complex educational perspective that John Dewey was to champion as progressivism. After Hegel, philosophy changed generally and it is no exaggeration to claim that all of the important developments in later philosophy represent an attempt to deal with the problems he highlighted and the system he posed and elaborated (Anderson, 1962).

Rousseau is said to have 'rediscovered the child' and 'rediscovered community'. Unsurprising in present times, as familiar as they are with developmental psychologies, Rousseau reminded his times that children were not merely 'little adults', that is, not like adults in thought, feeling and motives, just less able to act on them. Rather, they were quite different beings incapable of certain types of thought and judgement. He wrote a theory of education highlighting experiences that were appropriate and inappropriate to particular stages of a child's development. He forced a reconstrual of the child and childhood that had repercussions into modern times.

Equally, from his belief that all things are good as they come from the hands of the Maker but deteriorated in the hands of Man came Rousseau's criticism of society and an urge to recapture an understanding of *community*. In society we are individual units thrown together with little mutuality or shared interest. By contrast, community, as Tönnies (1887/1959) later differentiated it in his idea of *Gemeinschaft*, is 'all intimate, private, and exclusive being together', a state of being characterised by relative smallness of scale, commonality of interests, and cooperation based on something other than coercion; for example, on a natural cooperation within species (Kropotkin, 1902).

Hegel's thought is as notoriously difficult to capture succinctly as it is thoroughgoing and comprehensive. His ideas changed and developed over a number of years, but a theme running through all of his work and its developments is his concern over *fragmentation, divisiveness* and *particulars* in life; he framed the issue as that of *alienation*. Alienation signals separation and division, and thus there was a consequent need for coercion to force and keep these alienated atoms together in some sort of socially cohesive group.

Hegel's quest was to determine what conditions of mental life (mental outlooks or character structures) and of social life (forces or interests in society) create barriers between people and keep them alienated. The data that were history suggested to him that there was a detectable principle operating in human history, a principle that showed how an earlier stage of less adequate, less free, more coerced form of social life and social organisation gave way to a more adequate, freer social life and organisation. This principle was variously regarded as Spirit, Reason, Mind; whatever it was, it was over and beyond the individual.

This, then, is a brief sketch of the historical development of philosophy up to the appearance of two personages who represented a turning point. From here forward matters become much less easy to chart.

Developments

In response to Hegel's account of Mind and mind, of persons, history and social life, were to develop the significant perspectives that affect the contemporary philosophical scene in both general and specific ways. An indication of how the notion of alienation was dealt with by subsequent thinkers and systematic systems of thought indicates the range of Hegel's impact. For Marx (1844a), for example, alienation was explained in terms of production. The coercion of labour, particularly the specialisation of labour, generated a separation from one's labour *power* and the *product* of one's labour, forcing one to relate to *others* by means of what each could acquire with money (the wages exchanged for one's labour power), and it placed one in a position of not being able to act out the essential nature, the *essence*, of being human in free, productive activity. For existentialism, on the other hand, alienation lay in the fact of our interaction with others always being based on our 'objectification' of them, our efforts to turn them to being first and foremost objects for our use. We were born alienated and doomed to our own unique, subjective outlook on life. Yet, ironically, it was only through encounters with others that we could grow in our own authenticity and achieve that objectivity for which we all strive (Shearson, 1980). Again, for the anarchists, alienation resided in our giving up our sovereignty over our selves, the too easy acceptance of a position of subordination, of the legitimacy of *de jure* authority, especially when sovereignty and superordination is claimed by an institution as large and as potentially influential and pervasive as the State (Woodcock, 1986). For fascism, the reverse was the case. Alienation resides rather in our failure to see how the State was in reality the embodiment of supra-human qualities and only in and through the State did we amount to anything and did we overcome separation and the sense of isolation and powerlessness that was alienation. Indeed, the term 'fascism' comes from the Italian *fascio* of *fasces*, a bundle of sticks signifying strength in union, weakness in division.

Perhaps the two most significant of these last developments for later philosophy were Marxism and existentialism, two complex philosophical perspectives that have vied for dominance throughout the twentieth century. Marx argued, and contrary to Hegel's idealism that saw history as a history of ideas, that individuals are infinitely malleable and merely victims of socio-economic life, of the material conditions of their existence. Hence, Marx's famous dictum: it is not consciousness that determines life, but life that determines consciousness. Yet, to add to the ambiguities of Marxism, he was also to note that consciousness can 'act back' on those material conditions of life. Thus does Marxism lend itself to internal divisions between voluntarist and determinist readings. That is, we are sometimes held to be able to do something about our circumstances, at other times powerless in a world in which all is determined by forces we cannot influence or control. However, Marxism finds itself without a worked-out understanding of the individual, a worked-out *psychology*, and also without a theory of personality; two deficiencies that some have sought to remedy (Sève, 1974/1978; Leonard, 1984).

Existentialism, in contrast to Marxism, focused on the individual, and was more interested in the subjective experience of those same material conditions Marx had so forcefully centred in human life. Existentialism was more prepared to allow for greater significance to be placed on individual interpretation of those material conditions, how they were felt and understood by different individuals. The existentialists placed greater stress on the individual's 'lived world' and how the 'whole' was frequently greater than the sum of the parts of that lived world. In the slogan with which they became generally associated, that is, 'existence precedes essence', they insisted that there is no pre-given essence of human beings but rather any essence we might be able to discover always comes after the event, it grows out of lived experience, out of existence, out of what human beings are observed to do in the world.

These developments have impacted on all subsequent political thinking, but also on our conceptions of what counts as real or true education, on our theories in psychology, and our thinking in psychiatry, and so on. Bubner (1981) saw a renaissance of studies of Hegel's work well over a decade ago and historical-political crises of the past ten years may strengthen this as scholars go back to reconsider the origins of the ideas that have dominated the thought of the last century. This may become more pertinent as the difficulties or shortcomings inherent in more recent developments such as economic rationalism become more obvious and there is a return to theoretical issues focusing the big questions of humankind and society (D'Urso, 1971).

Two particular developments in mainstream philosophy of recent importance have been in philosophy of language and in philosophy of science.
Various issues and questions are addressed in the different though related
fields of linguistics, linguistic philosophy, philosophy of language, and even
theology of language. These questions and issues have ranged from syntac-
tical and semantic features of language and whether these are universal across
all languages, to questions of correct usage and the importance of *context*;
from the role of language in life and human consciousness to the apparently
very special position language appears to assume in the Bible. For example, in
expressions as in John 1:1 'in the beginning was the Word'; or in the power
given to Adam in Genesis 2:19–20 where Adam is allowed to *name* all living
things.

However these last questions are understood and whatever they provoke,
all of them are illuminated by a recognition of the socio-political context, and
of the constructive and constructing nature of language. Language is now
taken to be not a passive mode of communication, but the critical origin of
the way we construct reality and the way it constructs us (Floistad, 1981).

For Marxist perspectives, stressing as they do the significance of the material conditions of life as constitutive of consciousness, language becomes
intimately tied up with power. Just as the Adam of the Bible had a power in
the right to name all things, so the ruling class is said to maintain its power
through controlling language. Literacy is not mere word-recognition (functional literacy) but an exercise in which a particular consciousness is
constructed or deconstructed, an exercise which merges one in, or, alternatively, provides an outlet from the strictures of, a particular context (organic
literacy); it can be domesticating or liberating (Freire, 1972a, 1972b). The
ideological mechanisms through which reality is mediated and distorted have
become quite complex, but whatever that complexity, language is an important device by which a ruling group constructs and maintains its particular
view of the world, a particular view of the world that masquerades as rather a
'universal' view and one on which allegedly depends the whole of human civil-
isation rather than just one particular form of social organisation that the
power elite favours (Marcuse, 1964/1970). Moreover, this view becomes so
entrenched that it goes unquestioned, indeed, is unquestionable; it is somehow
just 'natural', that is, in Gramsci's (1965/1975) terms, a *hegemony*.

In the philosophy of science there has been an equally vigorous controversy. Since Kuhn's (1962/1970) provocative thesis on the nature of scientific
revolutions, the activity of scientists and the methodologies by which they
claim to work have been critically examined. This has led to perhaps something of a 'throwing out the baby with the bathwater' (Passmore, 1978), but it
has opened up important questions. For example, attempts to demarcate
science from what was not science (Popper, 1963), the question of the consequences for science of having to abandon the fact–value distinction (for
example, the Frankfurt School's development of the idea of substantive or
critical reason against instrumental reason), and the question of the

appropriate manner of differentiating what was an expanding from what was rather a degenerating research programme (Lakatos, 1970; Lakatos and Musgrave, 1970). Feyerabend (1975) entered the debate with the most radical, 'anarchist' position, suggesting that as science had in fact progressed by accident, trickery, good luck and ulterior motives to the pure pursuit of pure knowledge it claimed to be, then, as a temporary medicine at least, any and all research should be supported because there was no way of determining what was an expanding and what was a degenerating programme.

The Marxist perspective in philosophy of science forced a recognition of the manner in which the product of scientific endeavour, knowledge itself, was determined by human interests. Habermas's (1971) thesis, for example, was that the very activity we call reason, that is, what is to count as rational, is significantly influenced by human interests. What Habermas, and the earlier Frankfurt School for Social Research formed in the early 1920s, attempted to deal with was the fact of a value-laden science, and the observation that those values appeared to originate in a structured social organisation in which social class was the dominant organiser. Philosophy of science deriving from this perspective, a perspective which attempted to merge the ideas of Marx and Freud, drew attention to the problem of how the activity of science is perverted by an interest in *utility*, in the primacy of the criterion of 'usefulness' to some predetermined end of the activity in which a scientist was poised to engage. As the philosophers of technology like Ellul (1954/1965), Marcuse (1964/1970) and Heidegger (1954/1977) were to even more forcefully argue, the idea of science as inquiry, motivated by awe or wonder, gave way to a notion of technical problem-solving, motivated by concerns to solve industrial problems, increase profits or more effectively engineer social conformity and submissiveness. These last observations take us a little way from the classical Marxist perspective, though they convey well some of the core ideas of that perspective. More specifically to that perspective, Harris (1979) summarises the point in arguing the entrenched nature of the connection between science and social life when he refers to the 'structured misrepresentation of reality'; a misrepresentation he sees as most powerfully and thoroughly effected by the schooling system.

Existentialists had a different quarrel with science, especially when science was turned to a study of the individual or of the individual's intrapersonal and social life. Carroll (1974) calls attention to a tradition exemplified in the writings of Max Stirner, Friedrich Nietzsche and Fyodor Dostoevsky, a tradition he called anarcho-psychologism and which he sees as a precursor to the existentialist movement.

The three heroes of the anarcho-psychological tradition gave forceful answers to the question of what type of science might meet these last specifications. For Stirner it was not a science which let its concepts become reified as 'maxims', 'principles', 'standpoints', any of which concepts are 'fixed ideas' that form a 'wheel in the head' that controls the individual in his or her free inquiry. For Nietzsche only a science that rejected the cult of objectivity could satisfy these demands, a science which stressed *difference* rather than same-ness. For Dostoevsky, as science had circumscribed human capacities, only that science was acceptable which refused to blindly accept the faith that it was the unique determiner of knowledge:

> Dostoevsky continues Stirner and Nietzsche's anarchist defence of indi-vidual life as essentially unknowable, as flowing from a noumenal source which defies conceptualisation, as resistant to all equations. The rise of science has been corrosive of the free will manifest in this image, it has sought to make calculable and predictable that which is unpredictable. This science has progressively cut man to fit a Procrustean bed in which there is no space for wilful acts.
>
> (Carroll, 1974: 113)

Existentialism and phenomenology forged these themes into more thor-ough and more coherent positions, maintaining that link to human-social concerns that Hegel had reawakened in western philosophy in the mid-nineteenth century. The phenomenology of the later Husserl grew out of what he saw as a crisis in modern science, a crisis caused by the fact that the *Lebenswelt*, the life-world, had been forgotten as the origin of science in real-life questions of real-life people trying to make sense of their worlds. Husserl saw the crisis as an 'ethical' one in that science, as it had become, had jetti-soned these concerns as 'value-laden' and divorced itself from the everyday life of the individual to address ever more esoteric questions.

All of the foregoing developments generated a formidable set of problems that had to be faced by anyone staking a claim to their own position being 'scientific'. Both the social context and the individual dimension of subjective meaning-giving have to be taken into account, and in their interaction. These posed significant problems for philosophy which sought absolutes and 'foun-dations' for knowledge and conduct. A very real question is now that of just what science *is*; not purely an academic question, given that the claim to one's position being 'scientific' remains a powerful emotive one. Equally, the viability of philosophy itself becomes questioned as the full impacts of these developments are felt.

The revolution that Hegel provided the impetus for developed, then, a somewhat difficult position for philosophy itself. Despite the complexity of the foregoing developments, however, the fundamental questions of philos-ophy do appear to remain as Kant had given them: 'What can I know?'; 'What can I hope?'; 'What ought I do?'; 'What is humankind?' Certainly, we should begin by accepting these questions before preemptively ruling them illicit in the face of postmodern imperatives.

Domains

These last questions give us the main divisions, realms or domains of philosophy and others that grow from them as offshoots. It is of value to the present exercise of locating philosophy to remind ourselves of these domains.

Epistemology refers to the theory of knowledge, where 'theory' is used to suggest a set of related questions and issues, rather than as a general law or principle; as in theory of gravitation. Here, the classic quest has been for 'foundations', for some bedrock or basis for a claim to know something. Formal considerations have distinguished *knowing that* (propositional knowledge) from *knowing how* (procedural knowledge), arguing that there all knowledge claims reduce to one or other of these.

The formal matters aside, though questions of belief, evidence and truth are particularly important ones in considerations of *knowing that*, the development of epistemology saw two major responses to concerns to give an account of how and what we know: empiricism and rationalism. Empiricism holds that we know 'ideas' and we know them through sense impressions; *all* that we know derives from experience via the senses of sight, taste, touch, smell, hearing – and any others yet to be discovered. A secondary level of mental operation, that is, reflection, allows us to mix and match ideas to form more complex ideas. But the basic origin of knowledge is in the sense impressions that write on that blank sheet that is the mind; thus, the *tabula rasa* theory of mind. By contrast, rationalism, holds that at least *some* knowledge comes other than by sense experience. Pointing to common visual illusions that must leave us worried about the veridicalness of our knowledge claims, and to ideas that it is difficult to specify the sense impression for, such as knowledge of God or the concept of infinity, rationalists look elsewhere. Thus, *innate ideas* are postulated; we are born with some specific ideas.

Two perspectives have tried to mediate or compromise between these two grand traditions. One was offered by Kant, who suggested that all knowledge did indeed come from the senses, but that those sense impressions were preordered by the mind in a fashion that was invisible to us. Thus, mind imposes *categories*. We have our sense experiences in terms of an ordering we cannot escape; for example, we have those experiences in spatial and temporal dimensions that themselves are not given in sense impressions yet are an integral part of knowing the world. Yet, in privileging or prioritising the mind, Kant can be understood as offering but a version of rationalism.

The other attempted compromise perspective was pragmatism. This recognised sense impressions as the basis of knowledge and argued that a knowledge claim grew out of the use to which we wanted to put it, that is, the mind dealt with those impressions in terms of its interests. However, we were not free to make arbitrary use of those impressions as there are certain limitations imposed not by mind, but by the experiences themselves. As an example, given that 'axe' and 'feather' have their normal meanings, we are not free to say that a feather can cut down a tree; it just does not work. In giving priority to experience, however, it seems that pragmatism merges back into empiricism and represents less a compromise between rationalism and empiricism and more a particular type of empiricism.

This foundationalist approach to knowledge is critiqued by many of the thinkers of so-called postmodernity. For these thinkers, there can be no foundation for knowledge. In the very act of looking at the world for some bedrock of knowledge we are said to do so already with a 'gaze' that is pre-programmed. These thinkers see knowledge claims as simply dominant, localised paradigms, waiting to be jettisoned following a change in the power relationship in society, generating in turn the abandonment of a particular knowledge claim. The relativism of this position worries some, while others take issue with the general adequacy of the account of knowledge proposed by these last thinkers (Passmore, 1985; Scruton, 1994).

Metaphysics, too, emerges in two major perspectives or traditions: materialism and idealism. For the first, the ultimate constitution of the changing reality that confronts us is some sort of substance, or material stuff. For the idealist it is something other than a material substance: Soul is the most obvious response, Spirit or Mind less obvious but equally as forcefully asserted. Within this domain are subsets of issues: *ontology*, when the focus of the question of ultimate reality is that reality of the being which is human being, and the question raised as to whether a notion of *Being* might be sustained; that is, something over or more fundamental to my factual existence, my *being*. Or, when the reality under scrutiny is the whole universe and beyond, *cosmology* draws our attention. This last has found a resurgence of interest in recent times with the publication of such works as Hawking's (1988) *A Brief History of Time* and Davies' (1992) *The Mind of God*. More familiar territory, if no less vexing, is the mind–body problem where materialists like Armstrong (1968) claim a material basis for mind, essentially in brain, and idealists like Popper and Eccles (1977) look to some non-material 'ghost in the machine'.

Ethics is sometimes discussed in terms of normative and meta-ethics, though different terms are used by different thinkers (Edwards, 1972). The first refers to the justification of statements of a 'should' or 'ought' variety. The second is an inquiry into the nature of moral terms. If one follows Anderson (1962), then a perspective is offered which provides a useful distinction between ethics and morals. For Anderson, ethics was a science of the good, an inquiry into the nature of good and evil. Morals referred to rules of conduct and their justification. In the inquiry that is ethics, Anderson argued, we must look to mental activities, to mentalities or mental outlooks, to the way minds 'go on'; the criterion was to be internal coherence, self-consistency in that activity such that it was not self-defeating. His inquiries located three activities of mind that were inherently good: inquiry, love, cooperation. Their opposites, censorship, hate, and competitiveness, were evil because they were self-defeating and self-destructive, and represented a closing of the mind. Morals were a quite different matter, concerned with laying down rules of conduct which might in fact on occasion conflict with the type of mental activity Anderson had derived as a good.

Whatever the outcome of these arguments for distinctions between morals and ethics, the domain is a complex one. It is also as close to truly human concerns as one might come; what one knows or what one shares with others in terms of species-characteristics appears less significant than how one ought to conduct one's life with others, especially if one entertains a *hope* for the future. Thus of interest are two features of Broad's (1930/1962) classic discussion of ethics. One is that there are found to be five quite different systematic theories of the good; and he omits Hegel and Anderson. The other is his provocative conclusion about the nature of human beings and the impact of this on questions of morality and ethics. That is, the extreme complexity of the subject of human desire, emotion and action, and the 'paradoxical position of man, half animal and half angel . . . too refined to be comfortable in the stables and too coarse to be at ease in the drawing-room' (1930/1962: 284).

Logic concerns itself with the rules of valid argument. The philosophy of logic raises the question of whether logic, as a set of rules of thought, is somehow 'in' the world or in the human mind, is 'real' or merely 'psychological'. It brings forward certain formal rules of thought, such as the law of non-contradiction, and the principle of identity. It outlaws, or at least generates difficulties for, the so-called argument by analogy: because x and y have some properties in common, then they have all properties in common. Aristotle was the first to systematise these rules of valid argument and it is of value to note that such argument was frequently about ultimate features of the external world; for example the earlier arguments of Zeno about monistic accounts of motion as a series of motionless states, hence illogical.

Axiology is concerned with values, their nature, origins, justification and the nature of value judgements. Here are distinguished extrinsic and intrinsic values: value derived from the use of something for some other end (a knife for cutting) and something being valuable in itself (education, music). David Hume was an influential thinker in this field, especially in regard to the position that facts and values attracted different types of reasoning. Indeed, moral reasoning was not reasoning at all, and matters to do with values and morals were to be correctly understood as being about emotion rather than reason. Thus the emotive theory of value in ethics (where it pertains to the idea of 'good'), in morality (where it pertains to the idea of 'right') or aesthetics (where it pertains to the idea of 'beauty'). Similarly, value judgements would be seen as merely displays of emotion in that they commit a person to the belief that whatever is being so valued is good or bad, right or wrong, and so on.

Social philosophy deals with the determination of the best forms of social organisation for human beings or a particular group of human beings (for example, those living in a remote rural area in contrast to those living by the sea). Such questions as the following will be raised: Is there such a thing as human nature, and what do different conceptions of it imply for our capacity to have a life in society or community? What is the nature of 'the social' anyway, and to what do we refer when we say that it changes? Can there be a 'science' of society? How does a particular form of social arrangement relate to a particular form of mental outlook, personality or character structure?

Political philosophy is concerned with questions about the proper distribution of power in the social organisation determined as the best in the domain of social philosophical effort. Here, such questions and issues as the following will arise: the place and role of the State; arguments about social versus political revolution or reform; the role of history; development of concepts like justice, law, authority; and reviews of the various systematic political philosophies that have arisen.

Now, these domains of philosophy further illustrate the nature of this illusive field that is philosophy. It might have been possible once upon a time to work in a particular field and refuse to consider questions in another, charging their irrelevance to one's own field of interest. This, however, is no longer the case, confounding attempts to say clearly what philosophy itself is. However, in closing in on this field there is a final focus worth noting, that is, the modes of doing philosophy.

Modes

Finally, we might know philosophy through its methods or approach. Here, five such modes might be noted: normative, analytic, synthetic, speculative, critical.

Normative philosophy is an exercise in stating and defending particular values, standards, criteria. It most often takes the form of stating an 'ought' or 'should' in some domain and defending it. A good deal of old-fashioned philosophy proceeded in this way as a particular philosopher presented a 'philosophy of' something. Thus, philosophy of science done in a normative fashion might lay down the manner in which the scientific enterprise should proceed. The tradition of *the* scientific method is a case in point, the manner in which true or real science should proceed.

Analytic philosophy refers to both a process and to a 'moment' in the history of philosophy. As a broad, encompassing process, it refers to the dismantling of a problem into constitutive parts. A good example is in philosophy of education (Frankena, 1970) where the highest level of abstraction about what education is 'for' in a particular systematic normative philosophy of education will be critically considered. This will be considered alongside the similarly abstract level of factual belief about such matters as the nature of knowledge (its possibility or impossibility) or the essential nature of humankind (good or evil, competitive or cooperative). Then, in the same analytic mode will be disclosed the types of empirical, conceptual and historical matters that the normative philosophy endorses. Finally, the analytic approach will scrutinise the practical recommendations of a particular philosophy of education and review the whole system for consistency and coherence.

As a moment in the history of philosophy, a narrower analytic approach is identified in conceptual or linguistic analysis, the analysis of concepts or ideas to provide precision in their use. This was to come to a peak in the work of Wittgenstein, which drew philosophers away from the classical idea that words stood for things existing independently in the world, to an idea of language being like a game. Thus if one knew the rules one could play the game; if one knew how to use a word, then one understood that word. Analytic philosophy in this sense was an exercise in conceptual clarification so as to produce clear ideas. However, there was more than a little tinge of relativism here in that words and concepts to be analysed in terms of different forms of discourse and their coherence therein may have no necessary sense outside that form of discourse. Religion is a case in point for a position that might object to this. Religious claims might be meaningful within the particular field of discourse, but meaningless outside it; not a palatable outcome for a field claiming universal, absolute truth.

Synthetic philosophy is perhaps most simply understood as the opposite of analytic philosophy: putting together rather than taking apart. Synthetic philosophy combines ideas from different areas of philosophy to build systems of varying degrees of complexity. Marxism, for example, can be regarded as a synthetic philosophy in that it draws self-consciously on history and economics, and, in places consciously in other places subconsciously, on Hegel, Feuerbach, and Moses Hess. Existentialism, which might also be taken as an example of a synthetic philosophy, can be seen as a reaction to our inhuman treatment of each other which is used as 'data', and, then, drawing on psychology, on theology, on literature and history, a position is taken in respect to the general condition of humankind.

Speculative philosophy is akin to synthetic philosophy, but more adventurous. It is of an 'if–then' variety. For example, if b is true of our physiological functioning, as the biologists tell us, and s is true of our crowd behaviour, as the sociologists tell us, and p is so of our cognitive capacity, as the psychologists tell us, then a is our best hope, our immediate fate, or our best course of action under all of those circumstances. Speculative philosophers like to play with 'possible worlds' arguments, to raise questions like: what if there was a world where there were more than five senses available to a person? It can provide an overview of various fields of human inquiry, an overview which could be more satisfying if less verifiable or demonstrable. Voltaire's (1752/1967) tale 'Micromagus' is a witty example that illustrates what becomes of our efforts to explain everything when we speculate about how matters might look from the perspective of two visitors from other worlds. The views of the giant from Sirius and the dwarf from Saturn do considerable damage to our anthropocentric and value-free view of things!

Critical philosophy has several meanings, one contrasting it with a speculative approach which would identify the latter as more the work of the sage than the philosopher. Perhaps the best contrast here with the other modes is its use in the expression 'critical reasoning', devised by the Frankfurt School.

Critical reasoning, in its simplest explanation, attempts to go behind the 'givens' of a situation. Traditional reasoning tends to take a problem as given, or as it is given to us, and explores its solution. Critical reasoning asks the question: why this problem? That is, what other perhaps more fundamental problem am I being distracted from if I commit myself to solving the given problem? Traditional reasoning takes there to be a strict differentiation between facts and values, proceeds on the basis of a value-free science, and thereby misses the point of the location of that scientific activity in a social context which orchestrates these very beliefs and the problems presented to us for solution.

These modes of philosophy, characteristic approaches or methods, are not exclusive to philosophy. Indeed, the question of whether there is a distinctive method of philosophy remains a difficult and open one. Nonetheless, these modes of doing whatever one is doing, or has done, when claiming to be doing philosophy will figure somewhere in justifying the claim.

Concluding comment

These, then, are some of the central aspects in the history of philosophy, some of the issues philosophy has sought to deal with, and some of the recent efforts to direct it to fields, like language, that others think it should rather be rescued from.

We can know philosophy through its history, the history of the problems with which it deals, the types of positions that have emerged in response to those problems, the modes of approaching those problems. But when we attempt to discuss the philosophical dimensions of a particular development in another field, we are faced with the question: what is this 'philosophy' to which we refer?

The lessons of this historical and conceptual location are, then, threefold. First, different issues have confronted philosophers in different historical periods. For us, and for personal construct psychology, epistemology has been centred since Descartes, this being taken in recent times into philosophy of science and philosophy of language. Metaphysics has been relatively 'quieter'; though cosmology has had something of a recent revival. The era of the tradition that was more concerned with ontology, that is existentialism, is said by some to have passed (Charlesworth, 1975), though its core beliefs may be timeless (de Beauvoir, 1975; Shearson, 1980). Ethics is popular, though arguably appearing more as what we might call 'morals', and then in terms of practical problems as 'applied ethics'; charged by Passmore (1985) as even then being often little more than 'lay sermonising'. Social and political philosophy is not done in the precise manner or grand scale of Mill or Marx, but underpins much of what is done in other areas, not always exercising a benign influence.

Second, few formal positions even in philosophy have aspired to comprehensiveness across all of the domains. Plato is a case where this was so: Plato had a theory of knowledge and of reality, a view of ethics and morals, a theory of social organisation, of the distribution of power within that organisation, of the education of the young for life in that system, of the hope for a life after death, as well as a developed psychology. Hegel had a similarly comprehensive system, while others like Spinoza weaved comprehensive systems which reached into many areas of life.

The third point is related to the claim that personal construct psychology, like psychoanalysis – especially when taken beyond Freud to embrace such early thinkers as Jung and Adler – has a high degree of philosophical integrity. This is in terms both of its consistency with respectable positions within the wider domain of philosophy, and, from the opposite perspective, its capacity to provide the psychological element in more embracing positions that attempt to understand the human condition most generally.

With this brief background provided by the foregoing discussion in place, we can address the philosophical dimensions of personal construct psychology. As already signalled in some of the foregoing observations, we can expect this discussion to touch the widest range of domains of philosophy, and various of the modes identified as characterising its practice.

The point of the discussion here was to simply locate our primary interest – the philosophical dimensions of a particular psychology – in a conceptual and historical context. Many of the developments, certainly those post-Hegel, continue to themselves evolve, even when this means returning to the origins of philosophy in the ancient Greek world in one direction, or denying the very project that is philosophy in another. Nonetheless, while there may be differences concerning how the search might be conducted and what might be reasonably expected by way of answers, the basic questions framed so well by Kant remain.

2   Links and latencies

Kelly (1955/1991) names various individual thinkers and philosophical positions with whom or which he aligned himself or from whom or which he distanced himself. He does this first at the outset of his two-volume work in a quite specific though brief fashion, adding a series of sections that can be taken together as a longer discussion in the domain of philosophy of science. Elsewhere he admits that the philosophy and psychology of John Dewey 'can be read between many of the lines of the psychology of personal constructs' (Kelly, 1955/1991: I, 154/I, 108). Further, in various places Kelly draws sometimes passing, sometimes more detailed attention to such thinkers as Aristotle and a range of psychologists whose work went beyond a merely narrow or 'technical' focus to address issues of wider significance; such thinkers as Freud, James, Jung and Lewin, to mention a few. There were also references to narrower fields such as linguistics and psychodrama and the work of Korzybski and Moreno in these respective fields, chiefly in connection with therapeutic method. These last connections are taken up by Stewart and Barry (1991), though in respect of Korzybski we should perhaps note a less than favourable appraisal of his ideas by Roback (1964), an appraisal that lends weight to Leman's (1970) criticism of personal construct psychology through the linguistic theory to which it was initially aligned.

This said, it has been noted elsewhere (for example, Appelbaum, 1969; Holland, 1970; Neimeyer, 1985) that Kelly did not sufficiently acknowledge his debt to other thinkers, and frequently misunderstood, or at least did not give fair hearing to, theoretical positions that were quite consistent with and in fact usefully augmented his own. Existentialism is a case in point (Holland, 1970) as well as phenomenology (Warren, 1985).

Direct references

Domains

The first philosophical issue with which Kelly (1955/1991) is concerned is that of *epistemology*, where he identifies personal construct psychology with *gnosiology*. This is understood as the 'systematic analysis of the conceptions employed by ordinary and scientific thought in interpreting the world, and including an investigation of the art of knowledge as such' (1955/1991: I, 16/I, 12). This term, gnosiology, is less well known today and a likely source for the description is Baldwin's (1906/1960) *Dictionary of Psychology and Philosophy.*

What Kelly appears to be drawing attention to here is the narrower focus of gnosiology compared with epistemology, and, consequently, of personal construct psychology *vis-à-vis* epistemology. Whereas epistemology was concerned with the question of how knowledge originates, with the nature of knowledge, and the limits, if any, on what we can know, gnosiology looked to the concepts employed in everyday life – in both its informal and formal (e.g. in science) aspects – as a way of opening up the relations between our (psychological) efforts to interpret the world and what this tells us about the world as such and the possibilities of knowledge of it. Epistemology 'proper' would thus include or embrace, as Baldwin notes, a reflection back on the concepts we employ to interpret the world, these concepts being the focus of gnosiology. Baldwin goes on to distinguish psychology and epistemology, the former studying subjective states of mind when mind 'knows', whereas epistemology is concerned with the relation of thought to world, the 'subject–object relation which constitutes knowledge as such, and which is the presupposition of psychology as well as of every other science' (Baldwin, 1906/1960: 336). The relation between subject and object is the function of epistemology, and gnosiology is closer to psychology in this stable of activities.

This does not exhaust the questions we might ask about knowledge, and Scheffler (1965) has noted five different questions. The *epistemological* question raises the most fundamental issue of what knowledge is, seeking a definition or statement of criteria. The *genetic* question concerns the origination of knowledge and seeks an account of the process by which knowledge develops in individuals and groups. The *methodological* is the question of how we should best conduct the search for knowledge (for example, through introspection or empirical observation and experimentation?). The *evaluative* and the *pedagogical* questions concern what knowledge is of most worth or value for the purposes of 'transmission' and what are the best teaching methods for that 'transmission'.

In this last type of classification, personal construct psychology appears as more concerned with the *genetic* question, perhaps also with the *methodological*, rather than the epistemological as such. Thus, Kelly's identification of personal construct psychology with gnosiology is more deliberate than casual, and related to his focus on psychology rather than epistemology. It was also likely linked to the significance of pragmatism for personal construct psychology. Pragmatism, at least as it developed under Dewey, was more interested in the actual processes of thinking than in issues of what constituted knowledge and what were the criteria of a knowledge claim that would allow such claim to be distinguished from mere belief or opinion.

Within this now narrowed domain of epistemology, personal construct theory was *positivist* in the sense of the more abstract features of Comte's system, which system Kelly saw as being deprecated for some of Comte's practical proposals. What Kelly (1955/1991: I, 17/I, 12) means here by the more abstract and the more practical aspects of Comte's system is not immediately clear, but his positivist epistemology is clarified by identifying it with *empiricism*, particularly with *pragmatic logic*, clarified below. Comte (1848/1908) in fact discusses the social aspects of his positivism, indicating how it would likely not appeal to the 'governing classes' and how it implied significant changes to central political institutions. Perhaps these are the practical aspects to which Kelly refers.

Personal construct psychology is also identified with *monism*, in particular with *substantival* and *neutral* monism. Monism characterises a bundle of positions in philosophy but is generally a view in metaphysics that the ultimate constituent of the material world that appears to present itself to us is a single, unitary sort of 'stuff'; alternatively, it is a 'non-stuff', but, again, undifferentiated. Substantival monism is the view that what appears to be a multitude of different substances is in reality but one substance in different states or forms or from different perspectives. In turn, neutral monism, which is usually identified with William James and, for a time, Bertrand Russell (1927/1954), simply takes no stand on whether that ultimate constituent substance is material or non-material. In the form of the double-aspect theory in relation to the question of the relation of mind to matter, substantival neutral monism suggests that both mind and body are but different modes of presentation of the ultimate substance to which both are reducible; but neither is reducible to the other.

As suggested elsewhere (Warren, 1985), personal construct psychology appears compatible with either a materialist or a mentalistic theory, and aligning it with substantival, neutral monism may have been fortuitous. This said, and on reflection, it is useful to distinguish 'entity-monism' and 'existence-monism' (Passmore, 1973). Entity-monism refers to the view that there is only one real entity and the things we normally regard as different and distinct things are in reality but appearances of that single entity. By contrast, existence-monism admits differences between things but does not accept that things have different levels or orders of existence. In Anderson's (1962) terms, that is, there is but 'one way of being'. Personal construct psychology does not elevate any particular thing to a higher realm of understanding nor suggest that there are not independent things in the world. The particular significance of this will become clear when we consider realism and idealism below.

John Dewey and pragmatism

If the psychology and philosophy of John Dewey (1859–1952) can be read between the lines of personal construct psychology, then we should make an effort to consider Dewey's position in some detail here.

Dewey is identified as a *pragmatist*, the term derived from the Greek *pragma*, which meant 'action' and which is usually rendered in English as 'practice' or 'practical'. James (1907/1978) cites Peirce's introduction of the term into philosophy in 1878, noting the latter's explanation in terms of meaning lying in the practical significance of a thought.

Pragmatism is significantly associated with the work of Dewey and that of William James (1842–1910), though, as James admits, the term, in its technical sense at least, originates with Charles Sanders Peirce (1839–1914). James (1907/1978) characterised pragmatism as a method and a theory of truth. The pragmatic method considers a question or puzzle in terms of the practical consequences if one or other proposed solution was correct. As to truth, true ideas are

> those which we can assimilate, validate, corroborate and verify. False ideas are those we cannot. That is the practical difference it makes to us to have true ideas; that, therefore, is the meaning of truth, for it is all that truth is known as.
>
> (1907/1978: 97)

Peirce did not accept James' definition, and dealt with the disagreement by ceding to James the right to the term *pragmatism*, modifying it to *pragmaticism* as a descriptive of his own position. In broadest terms, however, the enterprise of pragmatism was from its earliest usage concerned to 'bring philosophy into relation to real Life and Action' (Murray, 1912: 70), and therein lies a dimension on which the originator, Peirce, and the populariser, James, can be differentiated. In summary form, this differentiation turns around James' focus on individual thought and thinking, contrasted with Peirce's focus on what is common or general in all thinking. As Gallie has explained, James, the psychologist, was interested in this or that particular individual's thinking, whereas Peirce, the philosopher, was interested in the essential generality of all thinking: 'language is essentially a vehicle whereby one expresses those parts of one's experience that *are* general, that must be "ours" rather than "mine" if they are to be communicated at all' (Gallie, 1952: 28–9).

From Peirce to James to Dewey, then, and via the sociology of Mead (1948), there is a development of that understanding of understanding that is pragmatism. Peirce's position was a position in logic and theory of knowledge; James' essentially a psychology. In turn, Mead's focus of convenience was social psychology, concerned with the broader picture, though related to the same focus of these other thinkers; that is, of 'individual self and consciousness in relation to the world and society', as Dewey said of him (cited in Jung, 1995: 672). As Gallie notes, quoting the North American James scholar R.B. Perry (1876–1957): 'the philosophical movement known as Pragmatism is largely the result of James's misunderstanding of Peirce' (1952: 30). In turn, Dewey was to adopt the term *instrumentalism* for his own theory, which owes as much to Peirce as to James (Gallie, 1952), but which synthesised ideas from each of these men.

Dewey's instrumentalism was elaborated in his discussion of the development of American pragmatism, where he characterises it as 'an attempt to constitute a precise logical theory of concepts, of judgments and inferences in their various forms, by considering primarily how thought functions in the experimental determinations of future consequences' (1932/1968: 26).

Now, in proposing to develop a compromise position between rationalism and empiricism, Peirce offered a new form of inference: retroduction or abduction, commonly called the method of hypothesis (Ackermann, 1965). This is presumably the pragmatic logic to which Kelly (1955/1991) refers. This is explained by contrast with *induction* and *deduction*, which are characteristic of empiricism and rationalism, respectively. While there are different types of the form of argument that is induction, it is generally understood as operating by making a series of observations and then generalising from them to a claim about all phenomena under examination.

Abduction begins with a puzzle or problem, posits a solution which is in the nature of a hypothesis, then accepts that the hypothesis is stating a valid argument or a truth because it explains things most economically or usefully. Thus: An elephant is sitting on my car in the car park; if the circus was in town and an elephant had escaped, then the elephant on my car would not be surprising; therefore, there is good reason to accept that the circus is in town.

One significant problem for induction, and for pragmatism, is that there will often be various and different hypotheses that could be offered to explain the same puzzling phenomenon. A method of deciding which hypothesis to use is thus required, and while it was not proposed as a solution to the problem at the level of epistemology, personal construct psychology is a thoroughgoing response to this problem at the psychological level. That is, hypotheses are framed in terms of constructs which *assist the elaboration* of one's construct system. A summary statement of Dewey's instrumentalism (Morrish, 1967), is interesting in that it captures an essential aspect of personal construct psychology in these terms: 'Knowledge is never an end-in-itself, it is always a means; it is a personal matter, and each individual uses it for the purpose of adapting himself to new problems, new situations and new involvements . . . to find personal solutions to his daily problems' (Morrish, 1967: 110).

Now, Dewey's conception of philosophy places it clearly within the domain of everyday lived experience, and that is the domain to which personal construct psychology is addressed. A long quote from Dewey is instructive because it not only serves to differentiate his perspective from others but also to show its range and relation to personal construct psychology:

> . . . there was indicated a philosophy which recognises the origin, place, and function of mind *in* an activity which controls the environment. Thus we have completed the circuit and returned to the conceptions of the first portion of this book: such as the biological continuity of human impulses and instincts with natural energies; the dependence of the growth of mind

upon participation in conjoint activities having a common purpose; the influence of the physical environment through the use made of it in the social medium; the necessity of utilisation of individual variations in desire and thinking for a progressively developing society; the unity of method and subject matter; the intrinsic continuity of ends and means; the recognition of mind as thinking which perceives and tests the meanings of behaviour.

(1916/1966: 323)

From this passage we can see in a 'nutshell' what Kelly (1955/1991) means when he indicates the influence of Dewey on the psychology of personal constructs. He is drawn to a Deweyan pragmatism which emphasises the manner in which we human beings think and problem-solve. That is, his interest is in a psychological perspective rather than the philosophical perspective that was the focus of Peirce's work. In this, he focuses on the individual, as Dewey had also done in his work on education. Novak (1983) has considered the significance of this in terms of the implications of personal construct psychology for education; that is, the practical effort of inducting the young into social living, but with regard to their own personal constructions. This emerges in the notion of 'child-centred education' that Dewey championed, or in an emphasis on the child's 'needs and interests'. In every case, just as systematic inquiry grew out of the practical needs of everyday life – the 'life-world' – education was to be tied closely to practical projects, experiential learning and involvement in, rather than passive talk about, that world.

This said, we need to retreat behind the fact that Kelly (1955/1991) developed a *psychological* theory, not a philosophy or a position that set out to resolve the traditional problems of philosophy. Pragmatism and neopragmatism have been significantly critiqued as philosophy, particularly in respect to issues of 'truth'; more so when they deny the notion of truth. Scruton (1994) attacks neopragmatists like Rorty (1980, 1991) for their reliance on a problematic view of truth as 'usefulness', and for falling back onto the correspondence theory of truth. Moreover, Scruton's conclusion concerning pragmatism as philosophy, particularly as a position answering the epistemological question, would be disturbing for personal construct psychology considered as something more than a psychology, more than a modest attempt to chart our psychological functioning: 'pragmatists are just what their name suggests – wily casuists like Protagoras who, armed with a few impregnable arguments, can always accuse their accusers of begging the question' (1994: 107). We do not have to be overly sensitive to such charges if we accept that personal construct psychology has the limited range of convenience originally specified of it.

Latencies

We can now consider how personal construct psychology relates to the ideas of other philosophers or philosophical systems than those specifically mentioned or mentioned only in passing throughout Kelly's writings. In particular, Spinoza, ethics, Kant, existentialism, phenomenology, Vico and Vaihinger.

Spinoza

Baruch Spinoza (1632–1677) is a systematic philosopher who is variously identified as a rationalist, a follower of Descartes, a pantheist, and even a mentor of Marxist epistemology (Hampshire, 1951). Spinoza was much admired by Hegel for the magnitude of the task he attempted; that is, to give an account of the whole cosmos and the place of humankind within it. The description of Spinoza as a systematic philosopher is most apt. What he presented was a metaphysical system in which everything that exists is interrelated. In this system, human beings and their minds are dynamic entities interacting with other entities, including other human beings, and psychological, social-political, epistemological, ethical and 'divine' features of the world are all explained in terms of interconnection and interaction.

The affinities between Spinoza's ideas and personal construct psychology extend beyond these general matters. In this respect, I have elsewhere suggested that if 'cognitive' was to be understood in any more than a simplistic way, especially for personal construct psychology, then the work of Spinoza was most informative for such an understanding (Warren, 1990b). What was important in this regard was Spinoza's discussion of the emotions. This area has been usefully elaborated by Neu (1977), who outlines and contrasts the diametrically different positions of Hume and Spinoza. For Hume, emotions were feelings ('affects', 'impressions') with thoughts accidentally attached, whereas for Spinoza emotions had an inherent and inseparable 'thought component'. Spinoza attempts to detail how these elements fit together in different situations: there is no essence of emotion or of a particular emotion, rather thoughts and affects are related in a particular events; for example, no 'jealousy' in general, rather jealousy arising in a particular event or incident in which thought (belief, idea) will be important in both the determination and discrimination of that emotion.

In these observations, and to clarify further, Spinoza might thus be seen as a background figure in the tradition from Hegel to Husserl, and then into phenomenology, as an attempt to give some account of the structure of mind, an account that is freed from (has 'bracketed') the limiting, particular experiences of life, bound up as they are with problems of distortion and illusion. Spinoza also provides an account of mind that leads to the statement of a positive ethics. That is, ethical characteristics were seen as factual and intrinsic to life, not relative nor transcendentally given. Rationality, in turn, is bound up with a broader notion of 'mentality' and comes to be identified with the operation of certain clusters of emotions.

The basic concept in Spinoza's account is that of the *conatus*. The *conatus* is an endeavour, tendency, drive or effort toward self-preservation: 'each thing, in so far as it is in itself, endeavours to persevere in its being' (Spinoza, 1677/1967: *Ethics* III, proposition 6). An individual, particular thing is such only by reason of having a *conatus* and without this tendency to self-preservation a thing would not be a distinct thing but merely part of some other; without *conatus* all would collapse into a chaotic flux in which no individual thing would be identifiable. *Conatus* might be seen as a homeostatic process or a process serving an equilibrium in both an inner and an external world of change and fluctuation. In human beings, *conatus* is desire, and while it may be regarded as a basic empirical notion in some theories, in Spinoza it is rather this logical principle in the terms just noted.

Spinoza distinguishes active and passive mental states. Active states are those originating from within the individual; passive mental states are those which originate in contact with the external world: 'what one does' contrasts with 'what happens to one'. The passive emotions (passions) arise as frustrations or obstructions in the way of the operation of the *conatus*, and in so far as one is so influenced by external 'objects' one is not acting in accordance with one's own nature. In such a state one is neither happy nor rational. Active emotions are those that contribute to one's functioning as an individual (acting according to one's *conatus*) and are rational (in the sense of recognising their origin and course in the individual rather than in responses to the external world).

In Spinoza we have a model of the person or of the human mind as follows. To be an individual thing requires (as a logical principle or as a matter of logic) some notion of a tendency to self-maintenance, self-perseverance or preservation in one's being; this he called the *conatus*, which manifests as desire. Emotions which have their origin 'within' the individual, and thus express the individual's *conatus*, are active, and a correlated set of these active emotions involve happiness, rationality and freedom. Passive emotions arise when *conatus* is blocked or frustrated by external forces and a correlated set of these involve unhappiness, irrationality and submissiveness. Moreover, and related to a discussion below concerning ethics, the active emotions are expressed in 'sociality'; that is, harmonious social life is a natural consequence of each individual expressing his or her own need for self-preservation. The question is not one of whether individual good and social good differ, rather, when active emotions reign, social good follows naturally. Underlying all of this is a view of mind in opposition to Descartes's dualist position, with Spinoza arguing for a single substance having two attributes; that is, substantival monism and attributive pluralism.

Throughout Spinoza's systematic philosophy the concern is with mind as a set of interrelated aspects; mind in which emotion and cognition are not opposite aspects but complementary. There can be no distinction between cognition and affect because our mental state at any point, including when we are apparently involved in the 'pure enjoyment' of an emotion or in the deepest concentration when trying to solve a problem, involves both ideas and feelings as inseparable aspects of our mental activity. Reason is not opposed to emotion but is itself an emotional force that interacts with other forces and can affect the passions, which arise when we have adequate ideas. Thus, passions are thought of as transitional states to be overcome through the development of clearer ideas about their objects.

What, then, does all this signify for personal construct psychology? One answer is that Spinoza broadens our conception of mind, offering a coherent account that does not require, indeed that denies, the separation of cognitive and other functions. For the cognitive psychologist the image is of mind imposing some order on a world, which world provides through sense impressions, somewhat passively received, those data which become the content of the mind; no matter how active (or, as John Locke would say, 'reflective') the mind is allowed to be in its 'processing of information'. For Spinoza, as for personal construct psychology, mind is conceived to be far more proactive.

A second matter arising from these observations on Spinoza's ideas and their significance for personal construct psychology is the opportunity to consider another philosophical matter: that of ethics. Ethics, as noted previously, is at once one of the more complex domains of philosophy, yet also the domain in which most people have an interest. The impediment to psychology contributing to the debate here has been essentially in terms of that debate being understood as one about 'shoulds', whereas psychology is about facts, about what 'is'; and the so-called 'naturalistic fallacy' says that we cannot derive an 'ought' from an 'is'.

Ethics

Waterman (1988), after noting various difficulties with the different perspectives in moral psychology and philosophy, suggested ways in which psychology might nonetheless make some contribution to ethical inquiry. In general, it might provide research evidence that assists the validation of claims concerning how moral judgements are made, focusing on what people actually do by way of supporting or otherwise the theories of why they do it.

In respect to personal construct psychology, two matters arise in this field of ethics, one stimulated by the discussion of Spinoza, the other more specific and concerned with Kelly's ethical theory. These are different to Waterman's (1988) idea of psychology providing evidence, but are rather bound up with the very approach of personal construct psychology itself.

The first matter concerns the manner in which Spinoza's concept of mind is analogous to that in personal construct psychology. The same striving for self-preservation, the refusal to differentiate cognitive and emotive elements, and goodness conceived in terms of matters that are intrinsic to a mode of operation of mind, or of a construct system, rather than external to it, are all most illustrative. Thomas (1984) discusses Spinoza's position as background to the Frankfurt School's treatment of 'reason', particularly the manner in which both Spinoza and critical reasoning developed by the School deal with the so-called 'fact–value' problem. As Doniela (1984) explains this, what is really at issue is a matter of two different types of *theorising* rather than two types of *theory*. The same propositions and the same judgement of their truth and falsity pertain; but whereas traditional reason, under the dominance of technological imperatives, is essentially exploitative in nature, critical reason is non-exploitative. The social consequences of the style of theorising are quite different: one linked to selfishness and the other to a broad human interest in understanding the world in its own terms. Thus, Kelly's focus on the person as scientist, enlarging, expanding and elaborating individual and group understanding, has an affinity with a concept of an ethical life growing naturally from a particular outlook on the world, one which took the world in its own terms; that is, one which took the world in a non-exploitative way. Further, Kelly was quite explicit concerning the acceptance by personal construct psychology of *values* in psychology; here, the Frankfurt School's entreaties were misplaced from the very beginning.

The second matter is more specific and is dealt with by Mair (1985, 1989) and by Shotter (1975) in a general way, but by Stojnov (1996) in a more focused manner for personal construct psychology. Walker (1992) has also made some observations pertinent to this field.

Walker (1992) raised the question as to whether Kelly's *description* of the person as a scientist went further and in fact emphasised the importance, the particular value, of good scientific activity. That is, whether he was making or also making a *proscription*, a statement that human beings not only did, but *ought* to act as good scientists; certainly such a view could be gauged from some of his writing on therapy. Walker suggests that Kelly clearly favoured liberalism, pluralism and diversity in the way experiments with different options in life are encouraged. The outcome of such experiments was, in turn, evaluated in terms of the criteria of how it enlarged our understanding of 'the world and ourselves in more useful, more comprehensive, and perhaps even more veridical ways' (Walker, 1996: 262). What was 'good', then, is the scientist or person who tests theories, 'putting theories effectively to the test and venturing beyond the obvious' (Walker, 1996: 267).

Stojnov's (1996) discussion is more focused than the foregoing observations and starts from the recognition that Kelly did not develop a theory of ethics as such. However, Stojnov argues that there was sufficient in Kelly's work to discern the general look of a theory of ethics from a personal construct psychology perspective. The discussion here ranges over morality, moral construing and ethical theory – which, from earlier observations, might be held to be three different matters – and it highlights interesting points. One such point echoes our previous speculation concerning the link to Spinoza. As Stojnov notes, personal construct psychology offers a solution for the 'reintegration of a person fragmented into many' including into 'cognitive' and 'emotive' aspects of being (1966: 187), contributing in fact to the suggestions Waterman (1988) had made but now in a more grounded fashion than merely adding empirical research. Like Mair (1985, 1989) and Shotter (1975), Stojnov finds a moral dimension *inherent* within personal construct psychology in the image of the person it conveys.

Shotter (1975) had challenged the 'image of man' in psychological research, arguing for a change of the then dominant image. What was required was an image of a more active, creative, engaged or involved *agent*. Psychology was to become a 'science in which we try to understand the nature of the responsibility we can have for the behaviour of things, especially ourselves' (1975: 84). Mair (1989) related a similar image of human beings in a life of dialogue and discourse. In his account, philosophy was a 'moral discipline that is being conceived, not an ethically neutral commentary on *homo sapiens*' (1989: 257).

Stojnov (1996) goes on to cite Husain (1983) to remind us that construing is continuous throughout a range across so-called cognitive, emotive and volitional activity. And he draws our attention to the manner in which personal construct psychology integrates values into theory construction, much the way Habermas does with human knowledge understood in terms of human interests. He argues more centrally, however, that, despite quotations from Kelly's work to the contrary (Kelly, 1962/1979d), we are not dealing with a relativist theory of ethics. This argument distinguishes the *content* of what we might say, that is, the particular view of goodness in different historical periods, from the form or structure of construing. Preemptive construing and a failure to move through the full Experience, Circumspection–Preemption–Control and Creativity Cycles is not merely implicative for less than optimal psychological functioning, but it is less true to our nature as constructive beings trying to make sense of our worlds.

The Experience Cycle (Kelly, 1970) involves Anticipation (a prediction is devised), Investment (the individual gets thoroughly involved in the prediction), Encounter (where the individual is open to the event in all of its experiential dimensions), Confirmation–Disconfirmation (the original prediction is validated, or otherwise) and Constructive Revision (appropriate adjustments are made which provide a new prediction for a renewed cycle). This is a cycle in which the activity of construction aims at the elaboration of one's construct system, which elaboration is understood as a desirable thing, a feature of optimal psychological functioning. Circumspection, where we are open to all possibilities, Preemption, where we narrow or close on a particular possibility, and Control, where we determine to proceed in this particular way rather than another, for the moment, turns again around action in a world where action is valued over inaction. And preemptive construing involves narrowing in order that we may proceed to choice making in an active engagement with the world, but temporarily. The completion of these cycles, and the initial but temporary resort to preemptive construing, is understood in personal construct psychology as desirable, a 'good' thing. One searches for a 'best fit', for the construction which provides the greatest elaboration, defini-tion and extension of one's construct system. This *mode* or *manner* of construing that assists the elaboration of a construct system is understood in normative terms. This is analogous to the way that the existentialists, who are otherwise sceptical about moral rules, that is, about 'shoulds', establish nonetheless such things as *choice* or one keeping to the forefront of one's consciousness the reality of one's own personal death, as modes of ensuring a non-cowardly, engaged, authentic life, which is judged as a 'good'. Moreover, the centrality of our construing of others in our constructions of our selves again emphasises this inherent moral, if not ethical, dimension.

Stojnov's paper is a most suggestive one for the ethical dimension of personal construct psychology. It goes to confirm an affinity with the position put by Spinoza, and also by Hegel in his development of the notion of *Sittlichkeit*, the ethical life conceived as the individual doing naturally and uncoerced what is individually *and* socially good. In Anderson's (1962) terms such goods as *inquiry, cooperation* and *love* fit most comfortably with personal construct psychology.

Moreover, there are circumstantial aspects to note in this discussion. The location of personal construct psychology as a 'humanistic psychology' is one such. If we differentiate different psychologies in terms of how they regard and treat the individual, then personal construct psychology presents an outlook that returns integrity to the individual. The individual is understood, that is, as a *person* with all of the moral connotations that that term has; a being possessing rights and freedoms always to be treated as an end, not a means. In regard to treatment, that person is to be centred in a dialogue that enters into his or her inner outlooks on the world, what Sartre calls a 'journey into interiority'. This is to be entered with care and a sense of having been honoured by such an invitation. Pertinent to later observations concerning the social-political philosophical dimension, we might suggest that there is here the operation of an egalitarian attitude which is essentially moral in being essentially non-exploitative.

Kant

Kant is an alternative contender to Hegel to be identified as the pivotal figure in the history of philosophy. Redding, for example, takes Kant as ushering in the period identified as 'modern philosophy', though his central argument is that Hegel completed Kant's move and provided it with a way of dealing with 'intentional human subjects objectively' (Redding, 1996: 1). This was through a development of *hermeneutics*.

Rowe (1978: 16) claims that personal construct psychology is in a philo-sophical line from Dewey, Peirce and Kant in turning attention to the 'thought worlds' or 'microcosms' that each person carried within (1978: 16). This is true in a general sense that each of these thinkers tried to develop a compromise position between rationalism and empiricism, though quite differently. Mahoney (1988) identifies Kant as one of three major figures who provided conceptual roots for constructive metatheory. And Rychlak (1994) distinguishes a Kantian and a Lockian position in respect to the idea of *construing*, identifying personal construct psychology with the Kantian. In contrast to Locke, whom he sees as using a 'building up' model of construction – akin to the construction of a building from different materials – Rychlak casts Kant's position as using the term *construe* as meaning 'to interpret' (1994: 96). Fransella (1995: 44), however, records that there is a reference to Kant in an unpublished manuscript of Kelly's where he notes that Kant had 'concentrated his attention on the nature of mind before experience touches it', and that because Kant lacked interest in 'the part which experience plays' this divorced his philosophy from psychological interest.

The general link to Kant has to be made primarily in terms of Kant offering what appears to be a congenial epistemology for personal construct psychology. The Kantian epistemology ranges widely but it appears that two aspects of it are pertinent: first, the differentiation of *phenomenal* and *noumenal* realms; second, the role of mind in the construction of knowledge through the operation of the Categories – the starting point itself for what the mind does, that is, perception, is itself a matter of *interpretation* (Rosen, 1991).

In general terms, Kant's point was that as the mind ordered experience in terms of the Categories which the mind imposed, and could not resist imposing, then all that was ever known was the world thus imposed upon, the *phenomenal* world. The world as it really was, the *noumenal* world, remained forever unknown and unknowable. The other side of this view was that rather than our knowledge of the world conforming to the objective world we think we observe, that everyday world of objects is in fact significantly a creation of mind. This gave epistemology a subjectivist turn and represented a revolution in thinking about these matters. Kant likened this to the revolution Copernicus initiated by suggesting that it was not the sun that revolved around the earth, but the earth that revolved around the sun. Now, these views do appear to be consistent with personal construct psychology in that Kelly (1955/1991) accepts the existence of a real world, but considers that we always know this through the templates we impose. Thus, the Categories that Kant finds the mind imposing are analogous to these templates.

There are, however, some problems with too close an identification with Kant. If we can only and ever know a world on which our categories have already been imposed, then we have no ground for assuming there is another world beyond that world. That is, there is no ground for positing a noumenal world at all. More specifically, Kant's Categories are entrenched in his wider epistemology and conceived as fixed for all experience. The individual templates Kelly is concerned with therefore would have to be seen as additional to the Categories Kant has in mind. Indeed, the Categories that Kant discusses are not individual, subjective impositions but a general feature of mind as mind, and required by his own strictly logical argument concerning the existence of necessary propositions. They are of two different types, space and time being distinguished from the other twelve: three each of Quantity, Quality, Relation, and Modality (Kant, 1787/1964: A80). These are quite different to what Kelly understands by constructs.

At the more general level of critique of Kant various matters are raised in addition to that already noted concerning the 'two worlds'. A rehearsal of the attacks on Kant's position is beyond present interests, but a couple of points are worth noting for the 'flavour' of the criticism. One concerns the idea that the Categories are essentially subjective. There is no reason why what Kant identifies as having been imposed by the mind should not rather be a feature of experience itself, that is, is an *objective* category observed in all instances of a particular phenomenon rather than something mind-dependent. The stress given to experience by pragmatism illustrates this type of criticism. A second point concerns the account of the Categories offered by Kant himself. Seung (1989), for example, argues that Kant has in fact two quite different conceptions of the Categories, with two different functions, and with awkward relations between his early discussion and his schematisation of the Categories in a later chapter of his *Critique*. Moreover, the Categories serve both logical and generic functions, leading to further inconsistencies. In short, when Kant is taken in the standard way as arguing that the world of phenomena is constructed through the operation of certain a priori principles, this leads into an untenable situation that his critics highlight. However, it can be read as arguing that the physical world exists but *can only be* interpreted through certain concepts we construct for an understanding of that world. Thus:

> The physical world cannot be constructed by mental operations, nor do we have the need to construct one, because it exists on its own. But we cannot take a single step in understanding that world without performing the critical task of constructing our concepts and theories, whether they yield a priori or a posteriori truths.

> (Seung, 1989: 132)

The Kantian connection to personal construct psychology is, then, an ambiguous one, though reasonable in general terms. There is an analogy in terms of Kant's philosophical, and essentially rationalist idea of the mind imposing on experience, and Kelly's psychological, and essentially empiricist idea of experience being preordered by the individual. Yet, Kant's 'mind' and Kelly's 'construct system' are quite different: the one located in an attempt to derive foundations for knowledge, the other located in individual experience and a search for meaning. Thus, perhaps, Kelly's own apparent departure from Kant as a significant mentor (Fransella, 1995: 44), and the tensions others have noted in a too ready acceptance of the specifics of Kant's position (Husain, 1983, Ford, Hayes and Adams-Webber, 1993). This said, Kant does stand in a line of thinkers who addressed the contribution of mind to the acquisition of knowledge and these aspects of his work are not unreasonably acknowledged. Again, Kant's own exhortation to psychology to properly address the contribution of the imagination to perception, and to acknowledge the need for a function of mind that synthesised sense impression, is equally instructive (Kant, 1787/1964: A121). There is also another Kantian connection noted below in connection with the Kantian scholar Vaihinger.

Existentialism

Existentialism has been a notoriously difficult 'ism' to delineate. It represents to different commentators a philosophy of crisis, a reaction to humankind's inhumanity to itself, a theory of morality that, paradoxically, denies the legitimacy of moral rules. To still others it is a championing of subjectivity and of the isolated, recalcitrant individual, or, simply descriptively, a historical movement that died with Jean-Paul Sartre. In this last respect, Simone de Beauvoir's observation is pertinent because the interest in understanding the world that she stresses of existentialism resonates with personal construct psychology, which discerns that interest not in a few, but in all people, whatever the level of the questions they pose. Responding to the question as to whether existentialism was dead following Sartre's death, she expressed the view that it was not. This was because Sartre's philosophy contained key ideas through which we might comprehend the world, even though the adoration of power encouraged in contemporary society generated a struggle for such understanding. She remained optimistic 'that even in a period marked by man's aggression and his desire to dominate, there will always be, as there always have been, some men whose desire is to understand, to comprehend' (Charlesworth, 1975: 26); thus would Sartre's existentialism not die.

Shearson (1975, 1980) discussed the problems in attempting to satisfactorily characterise existentialism. He argued forcefully that unless some core beliefs, assumptions or characteristics could be located in thinkers traditionally identified with this position, then there is no legitimacy in using the term as an 'ism'. Shearson (1975) located two central themes to which all writers traditionally identified with existentialism are oriented. Later (Shearson, 1980) he developed these into a comprehensive discussion of what emerges as a substantial philosophical position. These themes were identified as dealing with ontology, and with epistemology, that is, with the nature of *human existence*, or being and its relation to Being, and that *encounter* between individuals through which the significant knowledge of the world is derived, respectively. These principles undergird a view of knowledge based on an essential involvement of subject and object, rather than their detachment. In particular, it argues that our knowledge of human existence itself can only be gained through this form of encounter. By contrast to all other epistemologies, including that of Kant which Shearson (1980: 346) correctly sees as still attempting to account for knowledge in objectivist terms, existentialism starts from a single contention: 'that [human beings are] primordially open to that which stands over against [them]' (1980: 346). This 'openness' means a preparedness to deal with the paradox of how finite creatures such as ourselves can approach an understanding of that which endures well beyond us. In other terms, how creatures well aware of and trapped or lost in being can reflect on Being.

In more social-psychological terms, Van Cleve Morris (1961) had summarised existentialism as a view of the human condition emerging from the preparedness to acknowledge the paradox between two central principles or facts of life. One is the fact that we are the most important elements and the central features of each of our own individual worlds, assigning absolute value and worth to ourselves. The other is that we count for absolutely nothing in the cosmos; our individual lives, Life in general, our individual and group death go completely unnoticed, and the cosmos as such has no interest in whether, how or how long we live, nor whether, when and how we, as individuals, die. Existentialism, then, attempts on this analysis to deal with the paradox of our absolute worth and our ultimate worthlessness as individuals. At a level of social or psychological research and theorising it emphasises that we must always explore the human condition from a perspective of a passionate involvement with the realities of life, which of necessity includes the inevitability of death, responsibility and choice.

A number of writers have specifically attempted to chart the relations between existentialism and personal construct psychology, either to disclose the tributaries (Holland, 1970) or to develop the theory in alternative ways to the superficially attractive 'cognitive' direction for personal construct psychology (Epting, in Neimeyer, 1985). If not the first, Holland (1970) is one of the earliest critical commentators on the philosophical dimensions of personal construct psychology to raise this link. He chastises Kelly in the now familiar terms of Kelly not having given due recognition to other theories and theorists, then goes on to discuss one significant consequence of this. This was that the tradition that was existentialism offered personal construct psychology collaborative insights of considerable value, yet these were lost in Kelly's (1955/1991) too ready dismissal of it. Holland argues that Kelly was a 'reluctant existentialist', that he had a limited understanding of this position which, like phenomenology, shared his vision of the human condition. Holland particularises his argument by tying personal construct psychology to the work of the phenomenologist Dilthey and the existentialist Sartre.

Butt (1997), following Holland (1970), discusses personal construct psychology as a species of existential phenomenology, and suggests another useful link to that tradition in the work of Merleau-Ponty (Butt, 1998a). He argues that both personal construct psychology and existential phenomenology share a view of the self as process, agree on the role and significance of choice and action, and agree on the situatedness of that personal agency that is involved in choice and action. Equally of interest was Merleau-Ponty's notion of 'sedimentation', that is, an idea or a set of ideas that become 'fixed' and constitute, in personal construct psychology terms, *preemptive* construing. Butt (1998a) describes sedimented beliefs as beliefs that demand the primacy, the correctness, of one particular outlook against all alternatives, and no matter how limiting or distorting that perspective is, it is retained against evidence to the contrary. From Merleau-Ponty's perspective, we overcome sedimentation by particular types of activity, by truly *engaging* in different projects in the world.

Butt (1998b) finds the thought of Merleau-Ponty useful in developing personal construct psychology itself along the lines of a phenomenological, as opposed to a 'cognitive', reading. Thus, he finds both Sartre and Kelly offering what for Merleau-Ponty would be an overly optimistic view of our capacity to change. Sartre would be taken as giving too great a stress to our reason and our will, while Kelly would be overstressing our ability to identify with our superordinating system and thus bring about subordinate change.

It is interesting to extend these observations into Merleau-Ponty's stress on 'the body'. Such an extension provides another line of development of the relationship between existentialism and personal construct psychology and catches also the important idea of pre-verbal constructs which are 'likely to deal with the self as well as with other people and inanimate things' (Kelly, 1955/1991: I, 461/I, 341–2). Merleau-Ponty's early work concluded in terms of the failure of most traditional philosophy and psychology (especially cognitive psychology) to grasp the importance of the body in human experience of the world. Bodily experience provides us with 'a way of access to the world and the object, with a "praktognosia"'; the body 'has its world, or understands its world, without having to make use of my "symbolic" or "objectifying function"' (Merleau-Ponty, 1945/1962: 140–1). For personal construct psychology, a pre-verbal construct is one which is used in the absence of a consistent word symbol (Kelly, 1955/1991: I, 459/I, 340). Such a construct, moreover, is likely to be part of the core system and used to deal with the self, particularly in relation to matters of dependency (Kelly, 1962/1979e). And dependency is arguably one of the earliest experiences of the body in the world of other but more powerful bodies, including inanimate things, and even the giant and awesome forces of nature or the artefacts of a technological society.

Butt (1998b) has followed this last direction, urging that personal construct psychology consider the utility of seeing the person in terms of Merleau-Ponty's 'body subject' rather than a 'subject with a body'. In turn, the idea of commonality would be 'primitive' or 'primary' to human being, and individuality something that was 'achieved'; perhaps through a process of individuation as described by other theorists and discussed later (for example, Fromm, 1942; Jung, 1945/1953; Barbu, 1956).

There is in all of this last development a further important point for how a notion of *self* might be elaborated. Through the lens of Merleau-Ponty's work there is a possibility of locating a 'postmodern metaphysics' that does not succumb to 'either the excesses of philosophical totalisation or sceptical negation' (Johnson, 1993: 54); neither a self as mere subjectivity nor a mere locus of discourse. Equally with the self's body, to which we do an injustice in seeing it 'as the handmaiden of consciousness, or when we ignore the body's intelligent connections with the world at hand in order to draw attention to the linguistic constructions of social structures . . . and discourse' (O'Loughlin, 1997: 24–5).

Now, while the foregoing commentators have seen direct and latent connections between personal construct psychology and existentialism, Soffer (1990) is not convinced of the tightness of the existentialist connection. He identifies existentialism in terms of the positing by that position of 'the existence of originatory experiences that antedate the beginnings of knowledge and belong to the . . . lived world of immediate preconstructed experience' (1990: 361). These last experiences of this world cannot be reconstrued and any negative or disturbing aspects of such experiences must merely be endured. By contrast, Kelly appears to argue that negative experiences can be reconstrued, and they do not have to be merely tolerated as part of some 'human condition'. This argument is drawn from Kelly's own observations, which Soffer admits fall short of Kelly claiming that all or every disquieting experience reflects the dramatic dilemmas of the 'primitive', 'preconstructable' world. It is bolstered by reference to Kelly's cosmology, and to his notion of hostility. As to the first, Soffer finds the idea of an ordered universe that is amenable to reconstruction, as posited by personal construct psychology, conflicts with the existentialist notion of us simply having to accept that world which in fact is more capricious. As to the second, which is related to the first, the experience of hostility arises from our efforts to force a validation on that which we have found already to be invalidated. In this, we must accept that it is our effort to 'exhort validational evidence' that accounts for our feelings, rather than 'the situation' in which we, like all of humanity, find ourselves.

Soffer concludes that when Kelly referred to differences between his position and existentialism he was making more than a passing remark. There was a more fundamental difference which lay in the contrast between the personal construct psychology understanding of the human situation and that of the existentialists; a more optimistic against a more pessimistic outlook on the world and our capacity to deal with that world. The former saw the human situation as presenting no limitations on our capacity to construe even what appeared to be mysterious: 'the murky existentialist understanding of phenomenal experience (the "inner 'inner' feeling")' (Soffer, 1990: 374), whereas the existentialists posited a preconstructed base level that set some limits on our ability to construe. While an adjudication on these matters is made difficult by an absence of a clear and accepted definition of existentialism, Soffer's discussion offers a significant challenge to the too ready absorption of personal construct psychology to existentialism, at least to the psychological dimensions of existentialism.

Phenomenology

It has been suggested elsewhere (Holland, 1970; Warren, 1985, 1989) that despite Kelly's (1955/1991) specific rejection of phenomenology, his position is most comfortably seen as falling into this tradition. Indeed, despite that rejection, Kelly sees personal construct psychology as arising from a combination of 'certain features of neophenomenology [and] more conventional methodology' (1955/1991: I, 42/I, 29). When phenomenology is elaborated in terms of its rejection of explanatory hypotheses, and of reductionism, as stressing understanding and meaning, as a *methodology* and a *standpoint*, the connection is clearer.

This connection is particularly apt in respect of the notion of mind shared by personal construct psychology and phenomenology. For the phenomenologist the view of mind as an abstract cogniser possessed of little bits of cognised content called 'ideas' is inadequate. It is inadequate as a concept of mind as is shown in a long tradition of philosophy critiquing it; and it is inadequate to the task of doing justice to the richness, variety and complexity of our experience of the 'lived-world'. It is, moreover, an unfortunate legacy from that tradition that in the proposition 'I think, therefore I am' inflated the cognitive and set us on the quest for its identification and detailing, a quest that is more limiting than illuminating if we are concerned with the 'whole person'. The phenomenologist substitutes a notion that there is no distinction between the mind's activity of interpreting the world and the sensations which come to us from that world; there is a 'pre-operative' way of being in the world, what Merleau-Ponty called 'motor-intentionality', the natural and spontaneous reciprocity between self and the world which is lost in descriptions of 'inputs' or information processing. Bolton captures well this distinction and alerts us to a point we will reacess in a later caveat (Chapter 6) and beyond:

> . . . psychologism studies the mind as though it could be isolated from its aim of realising itself . . . this is the defining characteristic of a great deal of modern psychology: it is the objective study of subjectivity that has forgotten subjectivity's concern for objectivity. Hence, for example we have a . . . psychology of thinking concerned only with the way subjects process information. Such investigations, regarded from the phenomenological perspective, will fail to reach the heart of the phenomena they deal with, because these phenomena are mis-represented by their being considered in isolation from the intentionality of consciousness – its work in creating objectivities that transcend our experience, though remaining rooted within it.
>
> (1979: 249)

Further elaboration of the fit between personal construct psychology and phenomenology is left to later specific observations and the general account to emerge of personal construct psychology as fitting most comfortably into that development of phenomenology into hermeneutics. This is not a neat fit, as a later account of the difference between psychology and phenomenology will indicate. However, there are sufficient points of contact to characterise personal construct psychology as a phenomenological psychology. More strictly, this is an existential-phenomenology; that is, a focus on epistemology and ontology as these relate to specifically *human* entities in the world.

Giambattista Vico

Giambattista Vico (1668–1744) was an Italian philosopher and social theorist who attempted to place the study of history on a firmer footing than then contemporary philosophy would allow. Significant among his ideas was the importance of *myth*, which was a powerful window for seeing into the world of past societies. While psychic, or individual, elements may well enter myths at a later stage – for example, we might note Freud's disclosures in this regard – myths represent a kind of 'pure understanding' of the world, the world as it is. Heidegger's notion of going back to the original (Greek) words which are assumed to be closer to the first attempts to 'grasp something of the world', rather than to impose on the world, provides an analogy. The original word for some thing or event was the attempt of early human beings to grasp and share what they experienced 'of' the world. In the shifts and changes and encrustations on language as it is overtaken by particular interests, less of the world and more of 'psychic interests' or psycho-social interests can take over. The expropriation of female experience through doing violence to words describing female experience is a more recent example. For Vico, the development of humankind's early life turned around the centrality of being able to live with each other, that is, *sociality*, which was a progressive elaboration of a principle of *justice* (Anderson, 1962).

Vico took issue with Descartes because of what he felt was Descartes's overemphasis of subjects closer to the rationalist's heart: mathematics and physics. More interesting here, however, is the distinction Vico makes in the course of his criticism of Descartes, between things that are *made* and things that are *natural*. We can only know the things we have made, and we thus cannot have that true self-awareness that is posited in Descartes's 'I think, therefore I am'; whatever it is we have in this 'awareness', is not anything like a scientific truth. As he argues, Descartes's 'clear and distinct idea' held by the mind cannot be the criterion of knowledge, but more than this, it cannot be the criterion of that mind itself. While the mind apprehends itself it does not make itself, and because it does not make itself it remains ignorant of the manner in which it comes to apprehend itself. While reality remains always unknowable in any complete sense, we are not, however, passive observers of the world. Rather, we mimic the Creator through experimentation in and on the world. We construct experiments to test hypotheses about reality thereby creating and re-creating conditions and situations which, because created by us, we *can* know.

In general, Vico sought to reverse the priority given to the scientific disciplines against the study of history, and to establish the method of study in history as valid as that used in science. He foreshadows a later development in social thought which was to distinguish the human sciences from the natural sciences (*Geisteswissenschaften* from *Naturwissenschaften*). The natural world would never yield its secrets, whereas the human world studied by history, being made by human beings, was understandable, and understandable in a more intimate, deeper way because of the investigator's own involvement in that world through his or her own humanity. Moreover, the basis of the study of human being in human history was in *language*, this seen in Vico's twenty-fifth axiom to contain universal properties: 'There must in the nature of human things be a mental language common to all nations, which uniformly grasps the substance of things feasible in human social life' (Vico, 1744/1948: 60). His interesting example here, one which displays his interest in the origins of language among human beings as a species, relates to the 'proverbs or maxims of vulgar wisdom' in which basically the same meanings are expressed by all peoples, despite the variety of languages and places in which they are expressed (1744/1948: 60).

Another aspect of Vico's work that is arresting for present purposes is his discussion of 'poetic logic', which drives home the different ways in which language is used and underscores a difference between logic and 'psychologic' (Schiller, 1926). In particular, Vico notes the widespread tendency of expressing things about the inanimate world through metaphors of the human body or its activity, metaphors which we have no trouble understanding. His examples are such matters as 'mouth' for an opening, 'tooth' of a plough, a comb, or a saw, 'handful' for a small number, 'foot' for the end or bottom, the 'flesh' of fruit, 'thirsty' fields, vines 'going mad', trees 'weeping', and so on (1744/1948: 116). There are clearly provocative matters here for the wrestle of words, things and meanings that Yorke (1989) was highlighting for the task and effort of personal construct psychology.

Anderson's (1960) assessment of Vico is also of interest. In a critical review of Caponigri's *Time and Idea: The Theory of History of Giambattista Vico*, Anderson underscores what he sees as the real value in Vico's work. He suggests that what was *new* about Vico's 'new science' was the view that we could discover laws 'in the human subject-matter itself, in its own drives or ways of working, instead of being laid down from above or, in any case, coming from outside' (1960: 172). The only way Vico's new science could be made coherent and intelligible was by reading these laws off the world in an empirical manner, as they were 'immanent' within the world not transcendent of it. This involved the adoption of an 'empiricist philosophy and the rejection of all normative and totalistic doctrines' (1960: 172), as, for example, appealed to by idealism.

The identification of Vico as a congenial theorist for personal construct psychology is indeed an important exposure for the philosophical dimensions of personal construct psychology. It was made early by Rowe (1978), who quotes from Vico's *New Science*: 'Minds are formed by the character of language, not language by the minds of those who speak it' (1978: 12), wedding this to a general account of the different modes of understanding that are expressed in language, metaphor and myth. The most comprehensive discussion of Vico as providing important conceptual roots for constructivist psychology is given, however, by Mahoney (1988). He concludes that Vico's particular contribution derives from the 'recognition that "knowing" is not a form of disembodied intellectual reflection but, rather, an active and embodied engagement with life's challenges' (1988: 16). Butt (1996) has pursued this type of thinking into a discussion of personal construct psychology, arguing that because of this engagement it is most usefully seen not as a cognitive psychology but as a theory of social action.

This identification does appear to be well made and not insignificant given the perception of a continued relevance of Vico's thought. Thus, two and a half centuries on from its publication, his *New Science* was being discussed and first-time English translations of his other essays being published (Tagliacozzo, Mooney and Verene, 1976/1979). Moreover, the relevance of Vico's ideas to contemporary thought was seen in a variety of areas, including philosophy, psychology, anthropology and sociology. His 'new science', that is, was a science of all human phenomena (Pompa, 1976/1979), and that involved two claims relevant to personal construct psychology. One was that our knowledge of human phenomena could be scientific. The other was that a science of human phenomena, 'because it is *human* science . . . involves an appeal to an antecedent, experiential knowledge of what it is to be human [and thus] renders its products more intelligible than those of any purely natural science' (Pompa, 1976/1979: 45).

Hans Vaihinger

Hans Vaihinger (1852–1933) was a German philosopher who developed the philosophy of the 'as if'. The German text of his major work was translated by C.K. Ogden (Vaihinger, 1952), a co-author with I.A. Richards, of *The Meaning of Meaning* (1923/1972), which has been suggested as a source of some of Kelly's own ideas (Warren, 1985). That work criticises Vaihinger for not paying clearer attention to the relation between language and thought, which was the matter their own volume addressed. Vaihinger suffered from a significant defect of vision which forced a career choice on him that he would unlikely have otherwise made, and ultimately forced him to retire from active academic work in 1906, when he completed his most important work (Vaihinger, 1911/1952: xxxiv–xli). His interest in inconsistencies in life and the world, and his praise for philosophies of pessimism and irrationalism, might have similar psychological origins in the paradox he saw in his own life. This point is not raised as a trivial one, but to note again the intrusion of psychological factors as we noted in respect of Weber's theory; so with Vaihinger's life. Thus we underscore the significance of one's own lived-experience and how this might impact on the theories one finds attractive.

Vaihinger begins his major work with a dissertation on *thought*, thought as 'a purposive organic function'; though the wider notion of 'psyche' as an 'organic whole of so-called "mental" actions and reactions' is his real interest (1911/1952: 1). His argument in these opening remarks is that psychic processes no less than the organic or bodily activity of the organism have a utility function. The psychic function is a formative process that in its own growth, admittedly stimulated by outside forces, creates its own tools for more independent action on the external world; chiefly, 'forms of perception and thought, and certain concepts and other logical constructs' (1911/1952: 2).

In passages resonant with constructivist ideas, Vaihinger outlines his view of the mind as appropriative of experience from the external world, assimilative of that experience, and constructive of and with it. His account of mind as an active process of accommodation is particularly interesting in terms of the issue of objectivity. The purposeful activity of mind is to develop perceptual material into 'ideas, associations of ideas and conceptual constructs' that form a consistent and coherent system among themselves, but also to do this in a way which is 'objective'. Accepting that we cannot know objective reality but can only infer it, Vaihinger cashes objectivity in terms of our concepts, judgements, and so forth, allowing us to successfully negotiate the world. A long quote from Vaihinger illustrates both the point he is making and the echoes for personal construct psychology:

> We lay most stress on the *practical* corroboration, on the experimental test of the utility of the logical structures that are the product of the organic function of thought. It is not correspondences with an assumed 'objective reality' that can never be directly accessible to us, it is not the theoretical representation of an outer world in the mirror of consciousness nor the theoretical comparison of logical products with objective things which, in our view, guarantees that thought has fulfilled its purpose; it is rather the practical test as to whether it is possible with the help of those logical products to *calculate events that occur without our intervention* and to realise our impulses appropriately in accordance with the direction of the logical structures.
>
> (1911/1952: 3)

A core idea in Vaihinger's 'as if' philosophy is the notion of a *fiction*. A fiction is conceptually akin to an 'ideal type', something we know does not exist but which nonetheless assists us to orient ourselves to the world. Fictions can be self-contradictory, are accepted by the user as 'untrue', and they are not the same as 'hypotheses'. Hypotheses orient one to the real world, whereas fictions are supplements to any real-world understanding and represent an ideal world constructed in one's understanding.

There are further points worth making in respect of Vaihinger. First, as a student of Kant's philosophy, Vaihinger would have known Kant's (1787/1964) *antinomies*, that is, propositions which experience shows are equally defensible, yet which are contradictory. There are four of these situations where our reason is faced with a fundamental problem in advancing human knowledge. These four are: whether the world is or is not infinite in space and time; whether there are or are not 'simples', some ultimate irreducible elements in reality; whether there is or is not a form of causality outside the realm of nature, that is, freedom; and, whether or not the world has a 'first cause' (Kant, 1787/1964: A426–60).

In opting for one or other side of the antinomy we construct a 'fiction', and the sciences no less than philosophy are deeply engaged in the use of fictions. As Vaihinger says of the third antinomy:

> We encounter at the very threshold of these fictions one of the most important concepts ever formed by man, the idea of *freedom*; human actions are regarded as free and therefore as 'responsible' and contrasted with the 'necessary' course of human events.
>
> (1911/1952: 43)

For example, despite all of the difficulties with the concept of freedom and all of the empirical evidence of how all natural phenomena – of which human beings are a part – obey laws of cause and effect, we judge moral actions and criminal behaviour 'as if' freedom prevailed.

There is here a different 'Kantian-link' with personal construct psychology. That is, it is less a matter of Kant's distinction between noumenal and phenomenal worlds, or his idea of the mind's imposition of categories, than his attention to some very fundamental contradictions with which the human being must ultimately deal.

The second point relates to some observations on the concept of *apperception*. The concept of apperception is acknowledged by Vaihinger as above all other psychical processes in its usefulness to the activity of the mind (1911/1952: 1). Apperception is an old concept, one used differently by those thinkers who find a use for it. Kodis (1896: 384) notes three types of apperception to that time: as an event which imparts clearness to representations; as reflective knowledge; and as an act of knowledge produced by two groups of representations. Generally, apperception refers to a unifying and ordering element of mind. It finds its first formal expression in philosophy in Leibniz, who distinguished *perception* and *apperception*. The first, perception, is the simple representation of the external world in the inner world of the mind. The second, apperception, is the mind's conscious reflection on the inner state of that mind. Kant (1787/1964: A106–7) distinguished empirical and transcendental apperception. The first was the individual's awareness of his or her own state of consciousness at any particular time. The second was 'pure reason', the inner unchangeable fundamental unity of consciousness.

It was in Herbart's philosophy and psychology, however, that the term became better known, wedded as it was to his more practical approach and interest in education. For Herbart (1834/1891, 1806/1977) apperception was conceived as a process of assimilating the mass of sense experiences that filled the mind – a mass that was composed in part of contradictions and incomplete or vague ideas – to some sort of order or system with which new experiences are dealt with. The mind was conceived of as an active unity, and the creative activity of mind that was apperception was conceived as a kind of 'mental breathing', as natural and inherent to the organism as was physical breathing.

In his educational theory Herbart stressed that a teacher must always strive to ensure that any new material was presented to the pupil in a fashion that it could easily be integrated with what the child already knew. His pedagogic principles involved four steps through which a teacher was constantly checking that a pupil truly 'saw' a new idea correctly. These principles became a teaching method that endured into recent times and continues to have merit. These principles required Preparation (stating the aim of the lesson clearly), Presentation (gaining new information from reading, dialogue, experimentation, and so forth), Association (interpretation, comparison and abstraction, of new material to old), Generalisation (formulation of a general principle developed out of the Association step) and Application (evaluating other situations or experiences – existing ones in the 'apperceptive mass' or new ones – in terms of the generalisations made).

These notions of how the mind handles the contrariwise nature of experience, and of apperception and its application to education as Herbartianism, are provocative for our theme and remarkably akin to the manner in which personal construct psychology understands what is going on when we try to make sense of the world. Kelly (1964/1979h) makes a specific and positive reference to Vaihinger. He notes that the latter's position 'has particular value for psychology' and that it was worth 'pursuing'. Thus he goes on to discuss Vaihinger's 'fictions', or 'make believe' in Kelly's terms, as an essential feature of science. This occurs when a scientist, acting like a novelist, makes an imaginative leap by 'entertaining propositions which appear initially to be preposterous' (Kelly, 1964/1979h: 150). It occurs when the individual is faced with something new, which generates discomfort and threat, and resorts to framing a hypothesis and acting on it 'as if' it were true. Most generally of all, there is a challenge to explore the proposition that 'we regard clinical psychology as if it were the purest of sciences' (Kelly, 1964/1979h: 162), a sentiment to which we will return in a later chapter.

Again, it is Mahoney (1988), whose discussion of the historical foundations of constructive metatheory is so valuable in placing constructivism in conceptual and historical context, who provides the most significant commentary on Vaihinger and personal construct psychology. In particular, his conclusion is that Vaihinger had 'summarily outlined the major features of contemporary constructivism . . . [emphasizing] . . . the active and constructive nature of knowing and . . . [laid] . . . the foundations of a theory of dynamic structural development with self-organizing features' (1988: 26). This appears a well-taken conclusion, one that gains strength when the problem of the 'antinomies' of experience and the continued need for some sort of organising principle of mind – as in apperception – are recalled from Kant and Vaihinger.

Constructive alternativism as philosophy

In reaching back to uncover some of the philosophical roots of personal construct psychology, Kelly (1955/1991) first draws our attention to the view of 'man', of life and the universe, of construction systems and the predictive nature of constructs, that underlie personal construct psychology. He then indicates 'the philosophical position' that is constructive alternativism. This is done as a straightforward statement in which he emphasises that all present interpretations of the universe are subject to revision and replacement. He also emphasises that choice between different alternatives is always available, and that no one 'needs to paint himself into a corner; no one needs to be completely hemmed in by circumstances; no one needs to be the victim of his biography' (1955/1991: I, 15/I, 11).

He then asks whether the position he has sketched is a philosophy or a psychology, taking Dewey's distinction as that between the study of forms of thought (philosophy, chiefly understood as *logic*) and the actual thinking of people (psychology). However, this distinction itself is rejected because in studying the former he suggests we will come to see the latter; and in studying the individual's thinking we will come to see that individual's philosophy, or how he or she represents his or her circumstances to him- or herself. Thus, what he proposes is 'neither a conventional philosophy nor a conventional psychology' but a philosophy 'rooted in psychological observation of man', and 'a psychology concerned with the philosophical outlooks of individual man' (1955/1991: I, 15–16/I, 11–12). Thus, he refers to constructive alternativism as a 'philosophical point of view', but disavows any intention to elaborate it into a 'complete philosophical system' (1955/1991: I, 16/II, 12).

Now, how these moves around 'philosophical points of view', 'a philosophy', 'a philosophical system' and a 'philosophical position' are negotiated will turn around traditional understandings of such expressions. In turn, they will feed from a conception of philosophy. Anderson (1962) argues that philosophy consists in inquiry into the way things are; it is a critical exercise of judgement concerning the world. The task is to provide a theoretical account of the general nature of things, an *ontology* or general theory of being that is wider than can be expected from any of the particular sciences. In Anderson's account, a systematic account offering the generality he has centred as the task of philosophy itself, logic is the science par excellence. As Armstrong succinctly explains this:

Speakable reality is propositional in form. The general form of reality is therefore given by the general form of (true) propositions. The science which studies the general form of propositions is logic. In logic, therefore, or at least in this part of logic, we are studying the general nature of reality. So, logic is the science which studies the general nature of reality. It is ontology or metaphysics.

(1977: 68)

The account Anderson produced in terms of these specifications for philosophy he termed realism, and he saw the whole history of philosophy in terms of the defence of the realist position against the erroneous and self-contradictory position that was idealism. The debate between these two positions was, however, not one between competing epistemologies, but between two basic conceptions of the way the world was. We will return to realism and to Anderson's realism below. At this point it is sufficient to note that the question of just what philosophy 'is' is not an easy one. From what has already been said it is distinguished from other inquiries, however, in terms of the 'ultimacy' of the questions it addresses and the generally abstract, that is to say, conceptual or theoretical, perspective it adopts.

Now, Anderson's is what we might call a 'hard-line' view of philosophy. It is, in its attempt to provide a thoroughgoing account of all that exists and in a systematic fashion that recognises flux and change in an interconnected reality, a position in the tradition of Heraclitus, Spinoza and Hegel. Such a conception of philosophy issues in accounts that range across epistemology, ontology, social and political matters, ethics and theology; all of the matters covered in Kant's fundamental questions of philosophy. Moreover, as with Spinoza, Hegel and Anderson, these matters are seen to be interconnected. This interconnectedness helps us understand those accounts which see beauty, truth and goodness as intimately related (Bubner, 1981).

A 'philosophical system' that Kelly (1955/1991) disavows an interest in developing is thus harder to come by than his somewhat casual dismissal suggests. Few philosophers have attempted to state a system, Hegel being the notable exception. As Anderson says of him: 'he aimed at completeness, at a comprehensive treatment of the totality of things' (1962: 80). For Anderson, however, there was a difference between 'a system' of philosophy which purports to present a complete understanding of the *totality* of things, and a 'systematic' philosophy which stresses an underlying principle which applies to all phenomena. For him, this systematic principle will consist of a *logic* which will be historical, but itself not changing with history (Anderson, 1962: 86). It is doubtful that a philosophical system could arise from the perspective with which Kelly (1955/1991) begins, even if we had discovered such intentions. There is, however, a systematic philosophy in constructive alternativism that stresses an underlying principle applicable to all psychological phenomena.

A less hard-line conception of philosophy is seen in Dewey's notion of philosophy noted above. Here the focus is on the activity of mind in the world as it responds to problems and obstructions. Thinking is prompted by puzzles in the face of which the human being searches for a wider understanding of the everyday, or a meaningful understanding of the unusual. Heidegger (1954/1968) would differentiate puzzles and problems, reserving the domain of philosophy for the latter, but in any event, philosophy in Deweyean sense is more less all-encompassing and ideas of 'systems' give way to a concern with processes, processes rooted in practices.

A 'philosophical point of view', another of Kelly's (1955/1991) expressions, is not straightforward and could refer to a general position one takes in respect to the world – a set of assumptions about the world – or, alternatively, to a manner of casting questions about the world. The first might consist in its fullest expression in, for example, a Christian or a Buddhist or a Marxist point of view wherein one expresses in shorthand way a background of more basic assumptions about the world in response to a particular question asked of one. Thus, in a discussion about abortion or euthanasia, say, reference to someone taking a Christian view would be understood to mean that in respect of the particular practices of euthanasia or abortion that person brings a relatively certain or fixed perspective to bear. The second, a philosophical point of view as a way of recasting questions, trades on the key idea of philosophy as *inquiry*, as critical investigation; as contrast with advocacy, for example. Advocacy pertains to the first sense of a philosophical point of view and can issue in the statement of a normative position. A philosophical point of view in this second sense is more likely to be found questioning normative positions and simply means *critical* in the dictionary sense of 'involving or exercising careful judgement or observation'.

Constructive alternativism is more a 'philosophical point of view' in this first sense of being a general position in terms of which all else is framed. It consists of a basic proposition which is in the nature of an axiom. Kelly (1955/1991: I, 16/II, 12) also refers to constructive alternativism as a 'framework' in which he proposed to erect a limited psychological theory. This strengthens an understanding of constructive alternativism as a philosophical point of view in this sense of a general position we take in respect to how the world is. In turn, he fills out this position by aligning it with other philosophical *systems*. Yet, by reason of its thoroughgoing nature as a psychology, its congenial fit within other more embracing positions, particularly realism but also, paradoxically perhaps, hermeneutics, it is more than philosophy in a colloquial or 'slang' sense of being a way of life or attitude to life.

We will have occasion to remind ourselves of the different tasks of philosophy and psychology, but one significant strength of personal construct psychology lies in its 'fit' with substantive positions in philosophy, and its statement 'up front' of a philosophical point of view. Thus it was thought better to talk here of philosophical dimensions of personal construct psychology rather than the 'philosophy of' personal construct psychology.

Arising from this last point there is the notion of 'theory' and its relation to philosophy. At least four meanings of the term *theory* can be distinguished (O'Connor, 1957). One refers to a body of related problems or questions (as in epistemology as 'the theory of knowledge'). A second refers to a conceptual framework that might be abstract and quite removed from practical activity; mathematical theory is a case in point. A third is a more common-sense meaning which contrasts theory with practice (not itself a straightforward concept) where it refers to procedures, precepts or rules pertaining to a craft or activity. The fourth is the more formal sense where a theory is a logically interconnected set of confirmed hypotheses.

Kelly (1955/1991) refers to personal construct psychology as a *theory* in the first and fourth senses, though he stresses the fluid, tentative nature of theories. Indeed, theories are *thinking*, ways of 'binding together a multitude of facts' (1955/1991: I, 18/I, 13). As Bannister and Fransella (1971) remind us, theories as understood in personal construct psychology are not 'notions' (as in cognitive dissonance theory), not 'dogma' (not something that directs how we ought do things), and not about some artificially fenced-off domain of human life or functioning (as in theory of language or motivation).

Finally, in the context of talking about philosophy and theory in personal construct psychology, the term 'metatheory' occurs. The prefix 'meta' is ambiguous and can be taken as meaning 'after' or 'behind' or, more usually nowadays, 'about'. Metatheory is theory about theory and is taken to refer to a consideration of the shared manner in which a particular phenomenon is considered by different perspectives on it, or by different people, working within a particular field. Thus, metalanguage concerns the language in which language is itself discussed, metacognition concerns our understanding of the processes of understanding in problem-solving, learning and the like. In this sense, philosophy itself might be characterised as metainquiry, that is, as inquiry into inquiry.

Now, these are not particularly important matters for present purposes, nor is our discussion particularly sophisticated here. Mahoney (1988) refers to personal construct psychology's metatheory, indicating by this the broad historical and conceptual framework of ideas in which it might be located. Metatheory in this sense might be closer to what is commonly called a *philosophical position*. For present purposes, however, a philosophical position in respect of personal construct psychology is taken to mean simply the axiom or axioms on which it builds its theory. The theory 'implements' the 'philosophical assumption', here, of constructive alternativism and in a systematic fashion (Kelly, 1970). Moreover, while it is legitimate to refer to personal construct *theory*, rather than to personal construct *psychology*, such finesse is less relevant here. That is, in elaborating the philosophical dimensions of personal construct psychology we are already according a greater status and wider focus that arguments for use of the term 'theory' press upon us. Thus, mindful of these subtleties, we consciously use 'psychology' not theory, and understand metatheory as 'philosophical point of view' or 'philosophical position'; nothing significant is implied in such usage.

Realism and idealism

In the history of philosophy, the various opposing positions noted earlier, the different 'isms', become difficult to clearly characterise. Kelly (1955/1991) characterised one of those 'isms' as *realism* and disassociated himself from it if it was understood as holding that we were always victims of our circumstances. As noted elsewhere (Warren, 1985), this was a rather simplistic view of realism and Kelly did accept a more sensible if still simple view that realism accepts that there is a 'real world out there'.

Now, there is value in here elaborating arguably the most developed realist position, Anderson's position recognised now as Australian realism (Baker, 1986). Anderson's (1962) philosophy is developed as a realist position specifically in contrast to an idealist one, and realism given what is seen as its essential meaning. This elaboration will test a closer identification of personal construct psychology with realism, thereby, amongst other things, providing some directions for countering relativism.

Such a view that Anderson's realism might be integrated with a constructivist psychology would not be welcome in all circles. McMullen (1996) suggests that Anderson was unhappy with phenomenology and saw it as inconsistent with his realist position. Thus, any location of personal construct psychology in the phenomenological tradition would be problematic for such a view. Maze (1987) discusses the type of psychology that might emerge from Anderson's realism in a way that appears more open to a notion of mind as striving for, for example, meaning. But, a contemporary of Anderson's, O'Neil (1987), points out, just as Kelly would, that Anderson's acceptance of the separation of cognition, affection and conation is problematic. Again, Mackay, who has has a more specific and vigorous criticism in terms of the treatment of motivation in personal construct psychology, also makes a separation between motivation ('desires, purposes, hopes, fears, and so on'; 1997: 348) or *conation*, and *cognition* in his criticism of Kelly's (1955/1991) constructivism. Mackay's position appears to privilege conation on a similar argument to that of Anderson (1962), who privileges *affect* when characterising 'mind as feeling' by showing the inadequacies of cognitivism and conationalism. One basic response to Mackay's position on this last point is to simply restate one of the counterarguments he acknowledges; that is, along the lines of arguing that a construct 'transcends or incorporates both conation and cognition' (1997: 352). His evidence for rejecting this is, essentially, that Kelly's writing offers little support for such a position. Yet, caught between psychodynamic and behaviourist perspectives, it is not surprising that personal construct psychology was expressed initially in terms which lent credence to it being a 'cognitive' theory; and then to several decades of defence against such a characterisation. However, in the present context, Mackay's (1997) discussion of realism is more significant, drawing as it does on Anderson's position. One response here is that which Mackay himself allows and which is acknowledged elsewhere in the present volume. This is that personal construct psychology is a *psychology* not an *epistemology*; it is an attempt to give an account of the way minds function psychologically. Indeed, on the point of the present discussion, Anderson's (1962) summation of his own discussion is quite illuminating and resonant with ideas that are quite comfortable with personal construct psychology. For example, he allows that mental processes may exist with the individual only later becoming 'cognitively aware' of them (as, for example, with subsumed and non-verbal constructs), and that nothing mental is simply passive (Anderson, 1962: 74). Moreover, 'the notion of a "dispassionate reason" rests on a confusion between the *objectivity* of the issue (i.e. the simple contrast between truth and falsity, occurrence and non-occurrence) and the activity of the inquirer into the issue' (Anderson, 1962: 78). Personal construct psychology is more concerned with the latter, though, following the logic of pragmatism, it is also saying something that illuminates our understanding of epistemological realism.

An evaluation of Anderson's wider position takes us too far afield here, but we might note that Anderson had in fact little to say about phenomenology, though he does reject *phenomenalism*. A development of his philosophy in that direction, and the location of a congenial theory of meaning which he lacked, may not be as unpalatable as McMullen (1996) suggests; Weblin (1996) has argued in this way. To close the matter here, however, we might say that what we are seen to construct in personal construct psychology is *meaning*; a meaning with which we negotiate the world, which world is as the realist sees it, but with respect to which our meaning might be 'wrong'. Alternatively, the significant difference between Anderson's realism and personal construct psychology might be seen as due to the former working in the domain of large-scale *epistemology*, whereas the latter is a more limited *psychology* concerned with *gnosiology*. The type of psychology that would emerge from Anderson's realism is, then, not unequivocal. Understood in some ways, it does not align overly comfortably with personal construct psychology, but critically developed there is less of a problem. That matter aside, there are significant points of contact, certainly sufficient to make a consideration of Anderson's realism worthwhile here. That realism in short, is characterised as an *empiricism*, a *positivism* and a *pluralism*; by contrast to idealism, which commits to *dualism*, *relativism* and *monism*.

Pluralism means an acceptance that there are independently existing entities; in contrast to monism, which argues that every apparently independently existing entity is somehow united in or through a 'common' other entity in which they somehow 'inhere' or whose essence they share. Baker succinctly captures Anderson's position here:

> Contrary to monism . . . there are real differences between things, contrary to atomism there are real connections between things, and contrary to both there is no ultimate simple, or set of ultimate simples to which *complex situations* can be reduced.
>
> (1979: 6)

Examples of such overarching 'simples' are 'the Absolute' or 'the one true Being' (Overend, 1983: 3), and, for present purposes, notions of discourses or 'language games' as 'ultimates' or 'fundamentals' would fall to a similar criticism.

Positivism refers to the focus on a real world of natural, material and human dimensions, each to be understood in the same terms; there is but 'one way of being' (Anderson, 1962). Another term for positivism here is *naturalism*, an insistence that we view the world in the terms in which it presents itself to us. Freud was taken as a good example of this in psychology because he offered an account of mind that placed human mind in the context of the natural history of human beings in which so-called abnormal behaving was not discontinuous with so-called normal behaving. By contrast, relativism confounds qualities of things and the relations into which things enter. Thus, a thing is defined as that whose nature it is to have certain relations, '*that whereby* an event happens; its hidden cause or hidden meaning' (Anderson, 1962: 238). This introduces an a priori principle or a metaphysical principle between things in the world which must rather be taken as they are; that is, objectively or naturally as part of the world of complex events. In particular, in respect of knowledge, we cannot characterise either knowledge or the knower in terms of the relationship between them: the 'relation between knower and known, implies that each of these is an independent thing, or thing with an existence and character of its own' (Anderson, 1962: 42). Comte captured this well in some of the words used to characterise features of positivism – 'reality', 'usefulness', 'certainty', 'precision', 'organic', and 'relative' (understood as 'historical') – which was conceived as a move beyond both a religious and a metaphysical understanding. Comte's positivism was rooted in practical life and had social and moral implications based in that life.

Empiricism is posed as an opposition to rationalism in terms of the *logic* of each. Empiricism insists on a single way of being, of occurrences in space and time. These are to be known and understood without recourse to ideas of levels of truth or barriers between types of things; for example, minds which are to be known in one way, nature in another, God existing in another realm and unknowable in this realm, and so on.

In terms of the distinction between entity-monism and existence-monism noted above, realism is a *pluralist* position, rejecting that there is some fundamental substance 'above' or beyond' things in the world of which (only apparently independent) things are but 'moments', appearances, effects, outcomes, and so on. Rather, there pertains an existence-monism (which Anderson calls *empiricism*), and which holds that there are independent things which interact with one another all in the same realm of being. As Overend (1983) clarifies, in respect of this last point, there needs to be kept in mind a distinction between logical and material independence in following Anderson here. Pluralism holds that there is logical independence, not that there is material independence; things interact, and interact causally on each other. Idealism, by contrast, in holding that everything is in reality but part of a more basic or higher level thing (entity-monism), has significant problems with independence, with individual things in interaction.

Moreover, Anderson's realism rejects the *relativism* of the monistic dimension of idealism. Idealism, by accepting existence-monism – the logical interconnectedness of all (merely apparently different) things – accepts that there are levels of truth and reality. Whatever appears to hold of this realm is merely apparent and at a higher or more general, usually more privileged, level different truths might hold. There is in this view the beginning of a confusion of *ontological* with *epistemological* matters; a confusion between what a thing is and how it 'goes on', and our view of it from this or that social or biographical perspective.

Bickhard (1993) has taken up a similar point specifically in relation to constructivism, arguing that constructivism, properly understood, does not entail relativism. He notes the variety of constructivist positions, claiming that some of these, particularly social constructivism (constructionism), that propose a form of social idealism give 'constructivism a bad name'. His argument is that those constructivisms that do issue in a relativism do so because while they start from the common point of rejecting a passive view of mind, they introduce an additional and questionable proposition concerning something operating outside or beyond mind. Constructivism as such represents a strong position in epistemology and one fully compatible with realism. One way in which those constructionisms that lead to relativism falter is in their reliance on the very historical record that they have ruled out as merely relative and groundless; it is itself on its own argument merely 'just another construction with no more logical claim to acceptance than any other' (Bickhard, 1993: 281). More than this, social constructionism is argued to fall back on an encoding view of mental functioning, and in cases where language is centred in the analysis there are 'papered over' problems concerning 'the ontological relationships between babies and adults, and the epistemological relationships among adults', especially in terms of individuals and groups of individuals or societies (1993: 282). Bickhard's argument supports a view of knowledge construction based on some sort of trial and error process in which the 'knowledge construction must be some sort of variation and selection constructivism – an evolutionary epistemology' (1993: 280).

Noaparast (1995) offers an account of personal construct psychology in terms of a sophisticated realism that goes beyond my earlier somewhat simple account (Warren, 1985). That simple realism was identified, correctly, as an ontological realism, when the more significant task was to derive an epistemological realism. Noaparast moves personal construct psychology past pragmatism and into neo-pragmatism and a sophisticated realism. This, he argues, saves personal construct psychology from instrumentalism, which, as previously noted, saw ideas as instruments with which we work on the world, the criterion of 'workability' being critical; the 'it works' basis of a proposition or theory being true.

Noaparast's sophisticated realism consists of four tenets: that there is a real world independent of us; that our theories (constructions) can account for that world; that fact–theory distinctions are unacceptable; that our true sentences correspond to the reality of the world captured by our best theories. He argues from these that personal construct psychology is consistent with the sophisticated realism so characterised, and that it needs such a realism in order to avoid instrumentalism. The outcome is that personal construct psychology is characterised in terms of this sophisticated realism and a correspondence theory of truth. This moves it beyond Dewey to a new conception of pragmatism, one which incorporates the pragmatic notion of *coherence* along with the realist notion of *correspondence*. The similarities between the tenets of this sophisticated realism and Anderson's position are noteworthy.

Stevens (1998) has also examined in detail the relation between realism and personal construct psychology. He provides an account of 'minimum realism' which is argued to describe Kelly's (1955/1991) position. Minimum realism, again, accepts the existence of a real world independent of our construals of it. We can be mistaken about that world, simple or more complex in our understandings of it, but it is always 'it' that we are right, wrong, and so forth about. Minimum realism is akin to Searle's (1995) 'external realism' in relying on no particular theory of truth. Both constitute a kind of 'background' or context for all of our intentional behaving that is made possible by this pre-intentional level of acting or believing. Stevens links this minimalist realism to a range of ideas in different domains; for example, to the backgrounding of understanding in sensibility as considered neurophysiologically (Hundert, 1995), or the emergence of the cultural from the natural (Margolis, 1978).

Stevens (1998) develops personal construct psychology as integrating Margolis's (1978) natural and cultural orders. Thus, the sense-experience knowing, objectivity, non-intentional or pre-intentional capacities, linear causation, nomothetic laws and naive correspondence concept of truth encompassed by the first, meshes with understanding as a second-order knowing, subjectivity, intentional capacities, non-linear causation, idiographic focus, and a coherence view of truth stressed by the second. The integration argued to have been performed by personal construct psychology produces a 'realist constructivism' in which truth is understood as a 'sophisticated correspondence'. Howard (1997) takes a similar view to Stevens, suggesting that constructivism and realism are not contradictory but complementary. Needless to say, all of these views find Held's (1995) understanding of realism unattractive in so far as at least personal construct psychology is concerned.

Further, Chiari and Nuzzo, in a discussion aimed at bringing some order into the field of constructivist psychologies, note that a 'realist constructivism' is a contradiction in terms in the light of their discussion of the different constructivisms (1996b: 178). Theirs is a most perceptive account of constructivism and is revisited later. However, their point in respect of realism is that approaches that 'claim the subjective representation of an observer-independent, "out there" reality are excluded' by their definition of psychological constructivism. Such approaches, they feel, are better identified with a 'critical or limited realist metatheory', rather than with a constructivist one.

However, we might recall Bickhard's (1993) observations and also Merleau-Ponty's (1945/1962) stress on the pre-intentional to strengthen the realist connection, and also align it with the pragmatic and hermeneutic traditions. That is, Merleau-Ponty provides a particularly useful focus on the *human* side of the natural order, and both pragmatism and hermeneutics provide a lucid account of the sophistication of the 'correspondence' between mind and 'reality' envisaged in a realist constructivism.

There appear to be two alternatives emerging from this discussion. The first is to accept that personal construct psychology is just not compatible with a realist position. To move in this way means that we have decided on what realism is; and we have decided on what personal construct psychology is saying about the existence of a world 'out there' and our knowledge of it. This is a difficult position because of the different understandings of realism that can still be argued for in a coherent way. It is difficult because Kelly does clearly accept a simple ontological realism, and his position can be argued to resemble at least a minimal realism (Stevens, 1998) and to a sophisticated realism that merges coherence with a modified correspondence notion of validation (Noaparast, 1995). Thus, the second move is given in these last observations; that is, develop an understanding of realism that is consistent with personal construct psychology

But why should we want to identify personal construct psychology with realism? The reason is that we want to avoid the charge that personal construct psychology is merely subjective or merely a relativistic position. However the argument concerning realism is developed, what is being defended is primarily that personal construct psychology does not suggest that any construction is as good as any other; even if other constructivisms do wish to argue that way.

This question of subjectivity was discussed elsewhere (Warren, 1992b), where the views of three thinkers were taken by way of defending personal construct psychology against a charge of relativism. These were Deutscher (1983), Barbu (1956) and Bernstein (1983).

Deutscher (1983) suggested the importance of the verbs *objecting* and *subjecting* replacing 'objectivity' and 'subjectivity' to capture the process, the activity; subjecting and objecting are things we *do*, not states we achieve. Objectivism and subjectivism are rejected as distortions arising from an attempt to escape from a real human engagement with the world. Objectivity was better understood as 'disinterested interest' (1983: 54); an interest in finding out how things work by reference to those things themselves, rather than with reference to how we would like them to work.

Barbu (1956) suggested a concept of objectivity in his discussion of the democratic mentality. He meant by this that in any situation we encounter we have the capacity to be and remain aware that we are governed by a variety of internal and external forces, and that it is this ability to balance the often contradictory elements of this complexity that displays the objective frame of mind. Barbu characterises objectivity in terms of the individual's ability to look at the world through 'the categories of otherness, multiplicity, and formal relationship' (1956: 77). The most important of these is the capacity to understand another person, the non-self, or the non-identical as having its own reasons for its existence within itself.

Bernstein's (1983) argument was that the problem of objectivity and relativism is overcome in *hermeneutics*. In this context, he discusses Gadamer's approach via the interplay between different concepts of knowledge: *episteme*, *praxis*, *techne* and *phronesis*. *Episteme* is theoretical knowledge, scientific knowledge of that which is universal. *Praxis* is practical knowledge, knowing how to act; not *practice* or merely having a skill engaged in by habit, but practical activity guided by 'theory' which grows from practice. *Techne* is means–end thinking, the calculative thinking that characterises most of our intellectual effort in life lived in modern advanced technological society. *Phronesis* is 'ethical know-how' or *prudence*, an ability to get things done by compromise between the necessity of particular action and the reality of universal imperatives.

Bernstein argues that hermeneutics is the heir to this tradition of practical philosophy and, moreover, is itself a form of *phronesis*. The anxiety concerning objectivity and subjectivity is then seen to grow from a context in which modern life operates under a *deformation* of practical knowledge. This is especially manifest in the fixation on *method* or *methodology* (Gadamer, 1960/1975). It is in one direction seen in a context in which the methods appropriate to the physical sciences are taken over uncritically into the social sciences, which thereby lose their essential element, that is, *interpretation*. In particular, we lose sight of our rootedness in a world which we appear driven to interpret and understand, and interpret and understand through *phronesis*, a balanced, 'prudent' interpretation or *construction* of meaning. However, this does not lead to a mere subjectivity, but observes the *context* of dialogue in communities with 'the Other' which exhibit a degree of solidarity and in which various degrees of interpersonal relationships exist.

We do not, then, 'just dialogue', we dialogue about something as the object to which we, with others, turn our attention in terms of our individual interests and, when this attention is most intense, because we recognise something problematic in the world. That dialogue already presumes a rich background of shared experiences that are necessarily 'objective' for the practice of dialogue. We must accept some degree of shared objective reality or we cannot be understood, and we must be understood and understand others to dialogue with them.

By way of summarising the earlier discussion I offered the following conclusion from these three thinkers. As individual human beings we seek to understand our individual and social predicament. In this striving, we are always 'interested' in that our striving is always for a purpose, is always *subjec-*

tive; by definition, we as individuals are never 'disinterested', cannot escape our passionate involvement in life. Yet, we do seek, and appear to need to seek, some degree of understanding that transcends ourselves, transcends our *mere* subjectivity. When we attempt to convert objectivity to objectivism, to claim a once and for all 'complete' understanding, we have subverted our own subjectivity and its quest for understanding. Thus, we need an account of objectivity that *arises from* our fundamental subjectivity and is *not the antithesis* of it.

In short, what was suggested was that while we may all commence with an epistemological, ethical and metaphysical subjectivity, we strive and can in part achieve, as individuals, an objective position. It is important to stress that this is a *process*, however, not a *state*; we strive for the objective position, strive for something beyond mere subjectivity. As Bolton (1979) had put it, we too easily overlook that subjectivity strives for objectivity, that the central question asked from ancient times was 'what does it mean to be human?'; the question looks for something beyond mere subjectivity.

Personal construct psychology can be seen as an understanding of human understanding that advances us in our 'objecting'. That is, we are helped to understand that and how we, and others, subjectively construct more and more meaningful systems in order to have a more objective understanding of who and what and where we are. Personal construct theory is not lost in *mere* subjectivity and not a relativist position. The philosophical connections Kelly (1955/1991) makes, and the corollaries he develops to elaborate the fundamental postulate, take matters beyond the merely subjective. He asserts that there is a world 'out there' and we are indeed free to interpret it. Yet those interpretations will not 'work' if they are capricious; constructs are tested or validated against experience in the world, especially experience with others, and 'one construction is not as good as another' (Kelly, 1970: 1). Again, Kelly notes: 'Constructs cannot be tossed about willy-nilly without a person getting into difficulty' (1955/1991: I, 15/I, 11).

To return to the main discussion here, the following points support the view that personal construct psychology can be held to be a realist position: (a) Kelly (1955/1991) accepted the existence of the external world existing independently of our experience of it (simple ontological realism); (b) he misunderstood realism when he explicitly rejected a characterisation of personal construct psychology as realist; (c) coherent accounts of realism are available which are highly compatible with personal construct psychology (minimalist, sophisticated or Andersonian); (d) personal construct psychology is not an idealist position when considered against a most thoroughgoing account of a realist position, indeed is highly incompatible with such a position; and (e) it is not merely subjective, but compatible with a notion of 'subjecting'. Moreover, if the realism–idealism dichotomy is to be overcome by phenomenology, that overcoming does appear to still privilege a view of an externally existing reality which we *interpret* rather than *represent*, and which, as said, imposes its own restrictions in and through dialogue,

dialogue which always has to be about some-thing. Husserl's exhortation to return to 'the things themselves' was a major starting point for phenomenology.

Concluding comment

What is expressed in all of the thinkers with whom personal construct psychology has been implicated, and the larger scale 'isms' that it appears to resonate with, is the focus of the human being's attempt to make a sense of the world, and a sense that does justice to the active role of the individual, albeit importantly in terms of shared understandings. That there is a world to be made sense of is not in doubt in personal construct psychology, but how ultimately the sense of the world we make relates to how that world turns out to be remains an open question. Moreover, in reflecting on the very activity of sense-making itself we are provided with a systematic way of understanding sense-making, which is itself a part of the world we seek to understand. The realist connection will likely remain controversial, as will realism in philosophy, and it remains to be seen whether and how phenomenology, particularly as it has developed into hermeneutics, will overcome the realist–idealist tension. As far as realism is concerned, the call to return 'to the things themselves' made by both Husserl and Heidegger appears comfortable for realism, whatever these last thinkers did with those things when they got to them.

There are clear affinities between personal construct psychology and the ideas of Spinoza, affinities which extend into the type of ethical theory personal construct psychology might imply. The Kantian connection appears a little more tenuous, but reasonable in general terms and perhaps equally as interesting in respect of a smaller area of Kant's work, his discussion of the antinomies. Existentialism and phenomenology are also reasonably comfortable traditions for personal construct psychology, though if particular theorists of the existential tradition are examined closely, then the fit might not be as comfortable. In respect of Vico and Vaihinger, the affinities are striking and Mahoney (1988) appears justified in his excitement concerning these thinkers and the manner in which they stimulated personal construct psychology. Kelly's preparedness to address philosophical matters was a commendable start for the articulation of the psychology of personal constructs, and the controversies he thus embroils that perspective in are to be welcomed rather than despaired of in the conversaton about ourselves that he promotes.

3　Constructivisms

While matters are more complex than this might convey, it is helpful to use *constructivism* for views that see our understanding of our understanding of the world significantly constructed by the individual; and *constructionism* for those positions which understand our understanding more in terms of social factors, even if that understanding of our understanding is not itself understood in similar way. Gergen (1985) prefers the terms *constructionism* and *constructionist* in order to preserve the link to what he considers the seminal work by Berger and Luckmann (1966). He identifies a number of assumptions which characterise the social constructionist orientation. These are the view that the world we assume we experience is in fact experienced in terms of a matrix of interpretive rules located, primarily, in language and communicative rules; that the terms we use to understand the world are social artefacts having a historical location; that the survival of a particular way of understanding phenomena is determined not by its inherent or empirical superiority but by the social processes which find it useful to employ; that the dominant mode of understanding impacts on other dimensions of individual and social life.

Social theory

Berger and Luckmann (1966) provided the most influential account of these last matters, one that finds that the construction going on is significantly a social process. That is, that what we take to be reality, our 'knowledge' of an external world, is constructed essentially by *social* forces in respect of which the individual is relatively impotent. To avoid philosophical reactions along the lines of questioning what was meant by the term 'knowledge', they recast their argument as being concerned with 'what passes for "knowledge" in a society, regardless of the ultimate validity or invalidity ... of such "knowledge"' (1966: 3). Their domain was that of the *sociology of knowledge*, but a special reading of this domain: a less philosophical one and more an empirical one.

The general concept of the influence of social forces on our individual and group thinking is given most insistent expression in Marx's assertions: 'It is not consciousness that determines life, but life that determines consciousness' (1845: 37). Elsewhere, however, Marx allows some scope for an influence in the direction from the individual to the social: 'circumstances make men just as much as men make circumstances' (1845: 26). This variation in expression creates a tension between a deterministic and a voluntarist reading of Marx; that is, the view that individuals cannot influence the course of events, against the view that they can.

The Frankfurt School was later to look to psychoanalysis to provide a psychology, something that for them was significantly lacking in Marxism; there was a need to understand some things at a more idiosyncratic level of individual functioning. As Marcuse was to quip: 'not every kind of trouble or problem someone has, for example, with his or her girlfriend or boyfriend, is necessarily due to the Capitalist mode of production' (1978: 69). Since the Frankfurt School there has been for a time, and most notably relatively recently, a significant effort to write a psychology that was compatible with historical materialism and which took adequate account of individual factors (Sève, 1978; Tucker, 1980; Brenkert, 1983; Leonard, 1984). Thus, while the general articulation of the impact of social forces on the individual is important, the awareness emerged quite early that something is 'left out' in that articulation.

While many of the constructivist positions overlap, social constructionism stands out as important here. This is because it is social constructionism that has most aggressively confronted the perspective that is personal construct psychology. However, such a confrontation is arguably misplaced, as well as representing a *déjà vu* of earlier debates. Personal construct psychology appears to already accommodate the more reasonable claims of social constructionism, at least in embryo, and social constructionism is itself not unproblematic. We take up the last point first.

It is useful to visit a criticism of what appears to be the underlying idealist philosophical position on social constructionism. An excellent positioning of the issues and an argument for a social realist position arising out of a critique of what he identifies as social idealism is Overend's (1983) defence of objectivity; an argument which draws on the philosophy of Anderson (1962) previously noted, and on an earlier (Overend and Lewins, 1973) critique of Berger and Luckmann's (1966) work. Overend signals the conclusion of his own analysis at the outset:

> For social idealism, because of what I call the *problematics of demarcation, incommensurability, ideology, interests,* and *value,* there can be no objective social science. For social realism, because these problematics, upon analysis, are spurious, there are no grounds for suggesting the social sciences cannot be objective.
>
> (1983: 2)

Overend follows a method noted earlier, which, rather than pitting social idealism against social realism, develops the inconsistencies within the former position; this is known, since Hegel, as an 'immanent critique', or dialectic. An immanent critique or philosophic critique works by showing that the position under scrutiny is itself logically committed to features of the position it opposes; here, that idealism has to accept principles of realism for its own position to be coherent. Rather than appeal to some independent source for corroboration against idealism, this critique shows that a theorist cannot avoid inconsistencies because he or she is denying in the very argument being used matters on which his or her own argument relies. The distinction between realism and idealism as philosophical traditions is taken in terms of the three opposing dimensions which allow us to characterise a thoroughgoing realist position. As noted, realism was committed to *pluralism, positivism* and *empiricism*, while idealism was committed to *monism, relativism* and *dualism*.

Now, Overend argues that social idealism fails in social theory in trying to *demarcate* different realms or levels of functioning; as in differentiating the social and the empirical or the social and the philosophical. It fails in positing that the different realms or levels are *incommensurable*; that is, that there is a relativism between cultures, or between scientific paradigms. The socialising of philosophy and the claim that epistemology is dependent on social theory, as argued by Habermas, for example, fares no better; nor does Kuhn's conceptualisation of a paradigm as an ideology. Habermas is found to be on slightly better ground when he argues the role of interests, but he is said to elevate interests to too high, too rationalistic, a status such that they emerge as some sort of transcendental force rather than just another feature of the world. As Baker has it, 'the root of the trouble is rationalism – the attempt to find certain ultimates, certain identities from which a whole theoretical system will flow' (1986: 18). Finally, Overend argues against the fact–value dichotomy used by social idealists to bolster their case against objectivity in social theory. Here, he again develops Anderson's notion of ethics as a science just like the sciences of psychology and sociology. Ethical problems become just another feature of the world for the realist, whereas for the idealist they operate somehow differently, somehow in another realm; thus, again, for the idealist objectivity is rejected, but for the realist it is retained.

One might expand these observations concerning the problems for large-scale social theories for explanation in the social and behavioural sciences. One such problem raised against the Marxist analysis was in terms of the notion of causation it implied. In regard to the matter of causation, Aristotle distinguished four causes: (i) material, (ii) formal, (iii) efficient and (iv) final. The first, in the example of a house, say, is the material used; the timber and so forth with which it is built. The second is the plan that is to be followed in the construction, the detailed instructions on how to erect the building. The third is the builder who makes the house with that material and plan. The fourth is the end or purpose, the function intended to be performed by the building.

However, any discussion of cause must consider a second matter, a further important variable. This is the *field* in which a cause and an effect are identified. When the matter is approached in terms of the production of this or that effect by this or that cause, what is omitted from consideration is the field or context in which the alleged cause produces its alleged effect. What is in one context a necessary and sufficient cause may be in another neither necessary nor sufficient. Anderson elaborates:

> ... the fact that A cannot, as we say, make a Y become B, is nothing against it having that effect on an X and suggests no variability in the causation of B in the field X. Thus, what makes me angry may leave you quite indifferent, but this does not mean that there are not perfectly definite conditions of the occurrence of anger in me. Further, it does not mean that here are not definite conditions of the occurrence of anger in *men*; for what is necessary and sufficient for its occurrence in this wider field must be necessary and sufficient for its occurrence in me, and in you, as part of the field, but what is necessary and sufficient for its occurrence in me may not be necessary and sufficient for its occurrence in other men.
>
> (1962: 130)

It is not clear exactly how the social forces that construct the individual are understood, causally, in contemporary social constructionist positions. However, in so far as the position developed by Marx is a prototype for such positions, the question occurs as to whether the same problem of causation arises. Kamenka (1965) had seen this problem in Marxism, illustrating it by noting that the steam-mill may produce capitalism in certain social situations but would not necessarily do so in others. Thus he goes on to note how in Marx the social determinant ends up being given as 'the "entire" (never exhaustively specifiable) social situation' (1965: 102). Again, in regard to this prototype, Kolakowski (1971) had noted that even if Marx is not taken to be arguing that conscious intentions and thoughts of individuals were but a by-product of history, there is still scope for argument as to the role of free action in the historical process. While these observations can serve as no more than an interesting analogy here, it is interesting to consider social constructionism in the same critical terms as Marxism was considered in earlier times. These observations merely suggest that social constructionism, like Marxism before it, may be working with too simplistic a notion of causation, just as it may be committed to a social idealism that is self-contradictory and cannot be sustained.

As social theory, then, social constructionism presents a challenging argument and one that will undoubtedly unfold in different ways. However, it may be still subject to similar philosophical problems as arose for Marxism. This is not to say that social constructionism can be simply mapped onto a Marxist analysis. However, one is as equally struck by the obvious similarity of these approaches as by the relative absence of significant references to Marx in the literature of social constructionism. And this despite the fact that a major influence on its major influence (Berger and Luckmann, 1966) was Marxism.

Psychology

With these reservations about the underlying philosophical difficulties for social constructionism as a background, we can turn to specific questions of constructivism in psychology. Gergen (1985) reviewed the social constructionist movement in psychology. He distinguished an *exogenic* perspective from an *endogenic* perspective. The first flows from that tradition in theory of knowledge that identifies such thinkers as Locke and Hume and which takes the view that knowledge 'copies (or should ideally copy) the contours of the world' (1985: 269). The second perspective, associated with the names of such thinkers as Kant and Nietszche, as well as with phenomenology, is one in which knowledge 'depends on process (sometimes viewed as innate) endemic to the organism' (1985: 269).

In addition to the distinction elaborated by Gergen (1985), there are various differentiations made between different 'types' of constructivism. For example, von Glasersfeld's *radical* constructivism sees knowledge as actively built up as an adaptive function serving the organism's continued viability, with cognition functioning as an organiser of the experiential world rather than a discoverer of an external world (1995: 51). *Trivial* constructivism, meanwhile, is the simple notion that knowledge 'builds up' or accumulates from our action on sensory inputs (the power of the mind to 'reflect', as in Locke's account of knowledge).

Moshman's (1982) three types or paradigms of constructivism – *exogenous*, *endogenous* and *dialectical* – are less familiar but informative. These derive, respectively, from metaphors of the learner as a machine which processes sensory experience derived from the real world; as organism which has its own processes of coordination and manipulation of sensory inputs (again akin to Locke's notion of the mind's power of reflection, perhaps); and 'contextualisation'. The last is a process in which external and internal features – organism and environment – interact to produce syntheses which are not so much 'true' or 'truer' than any other, but which are simply 'more adequate than their predecessors' (1982: 375).

Steier (1991a) distinguishes between *naive* (first-order) and *social* (second-order) constructivism and makes possible the most significant distinction as far as personal construct psychology is concerned. The first, naive constructivism, is an attempt to keep the observer out of the research activity and to hold on to an idea of objectivity. This, Steier argues, is 'tautologically non-reflexive'; reflexivity having been earlier defined as 'a bending back on itself' or a 'turning-back of one's experience upon oneself' (1991a: 2), and identified as a vital component of social research. He also offers another type of constructivism, perhaps a subtype of social constructivism, in *ecological* constructivism (Steier, 1991b). This emphasises the smaller-scale 'contextuality' of, say, research, where, consistently with the social constructivist position, interaction between researcher and 'subject', and the alleged 'boundaries' between them, generates new understandings not available from each separately.

An identification of personal construct psychology as naive constructivism is implied in the stress on social construction, and this is more explicit in another contribution to the collection in which the last observation is made. This is Krippendorf's observation where he first contrasts naive and radical constructivism and notes how the former assumes that constructions are performed 'in response to a reality assumed to have a definite structure *outside* its observer', then charges that in

> accounting for the construction of persons in the mind of others, George Kelly (1955) avoids referring to that outside reality but, by failing to apply his constructivism to his own knowledge, he makes the personal constructs in other people's mind into external objects his theory claims to represent.
>
> (1991: 115)

From early on there was also interest in examining Piaget's constructivism in relation to personal construct psychology, some arguing a less (for example, Salmon, 1970), others a more fruitful connection (for example, Sigel and Holmgren, 1983; Soffer, 1993). An earlier point noted as a criticism raised against Kant's position was that what Kant saw as mind-imposed might equally have been seen as rather a feature of experience itself. This criticism accords, in fact, with the type of position taken by Piaget; that is, that *all* of our concepts are built up from experience. Whatever the similarities, personal construct psychology appears, however, to work with a more flexible and fluid notion of construction than does Piaget.

Mancuso (1996a) has argued how personal construct psychology and narrative psychology might be integrated with social constructionism. While Mancuso notes that some social constructionists did think that there were useful things to learn from personal construct psychology (for example, Harré and Gillett, 1994), Burkitt (1996) found Mancuso's argument lacking and, in fact, significant problems for any integration between the two positions. In particular, the problem was seen in terms of the different metaphysical traditions from which personal construct psychology and social constructivism emerge. What would be useful, Burkitt suggests, is an account of how personal constructs 'can appear within the broader framework of social constructions; in other words, how shared, socially produced text can be adapted and changed by social individuals in their practices' (1996: 72). Wortham (1996) also draws attention to what he sees as deficiencies in Mancuso's account, sharpening the disagreement as that over *what* is constructed and *how* it is constructed.

For social constructionists the better level of explanation is that of social and cultural relations in which individuals cannot avoid being involved. Mancuso (1996b), however (with a developing chorus of writers such as those gathered by Kalekin-Fishman and Walker, 1996), reiterates that personal construct psychology does not deny the social, rather it emphasises specifically the significance of interpersonal relations. Moreover, it does this in a way which offers, potentially at least, insight not only into the manner in which reality is socially constructed, but into the manner in which social reality is constructed (Searle, 1995).

In the intellectual climate that generates these differences of emphasis, Rychlak (1993) has proposed a 'principle of complementarity' by way of clarifying the differences between not only different constructivisms, but also different perspectives in psychology generally. He differentiates four theoretical groundings that might complement one another if proponents make it clear at the outset where they are coming from by explicitly acknowledging the grounding they are adopting. These are *Physikos*, *Bios*, *Socius* and *Logos*. The first involves an approach at the level of physical processes that are taken as no different between animate and inanimate entities. The second does distinguish inanimate and animate, looking to processes that are pertinent to the animate, as in the understanding of psychology as a biological science.

Matters get more interesting for present purposes when the focus shifts to the next two grounds. When persons are thought of in terms of their group memberships and the cultural influences acting on them, then it is the *Socius* grounding that is emphasised. Rychlak instances Gergen (1985, 1989a) as an exemplar of this grounding. Finally, when psychological theory is grounded in a recognition of 'patterned order of experience to explain things according to processes like prediction, personal construing, or mental acts in the Brentanoan sense' (Rychlak, 1993: 936), it is grounded in the *Logos*. Such a grounding focuses that cognitive organising principle that is *meaning*: 'To *mean* is to intentionally pattern or simply acknowledge extant organizations of experience that suggest a purpose' (Rychlak, 1993: 937). Elsewhere, Rychlak has suggested how his logical learning theory is well suited to a social constructionism of the Berger and Luckmann (1966) kind which 'views social norms, communal myths, and so forth, as predications held in common by people rather than as some kind of supraindividual (efficiently caused) "force in the sky" that patterns or shapes their behaviour in a mediational fashion' (Rychlak, 1994: 290).

However, his learning theory there being discussed, like personal construct psychology, is a theory of processes in the *Logos*. Social constructionism of a type that would deny significance to the *Logos* has to be recognised, but as complementary in the best case, irrelevant in the worst, to understanding of the *Logos* processes. Indeed, in the face of any such claim to the priority of *Socius* processes, there is the matter raised by Searle (1995) concerning how social reality itself is constructed by the individual; questions concerning the social construction of reality have to be aligned with those concerning the construction of social reality. Social factors and forces, interests and influences do not somehow float around in the ether capturing unsuspecting individuals and exerting some mysterious control over them. There is a related point here to McWilliams' (1996) discussion of the problems caused by the verb 'to be'. This verb effects an unconscious preemptive labelling in which some thing 'is' in some way, rather than being 'taken to be that way' by the utterer of a proposition. Thus we can make clearer attributions for propositions if we drop the verb 'to be' using what is called E-prime. We can then more clearly see that our propositions do not 'arise from the ether or lie under rocks awaiting our discovery' (McWilliams 1996: 71); that is, the locus is in us.

Elsewhere, Rychlak (1990) has specifically differentiated the type of construction envisaged by personal construct psychology from construction as envisaged by the social constructionist position of Gergen and Harré. In these two theorists he sees an old-fashioned mediation model of psychological functioning which leaves little place for agency or dialectical reasoning, and which cannot account for the behaviourist theory itself. The self in such views is merely a mediating process, 'a conveyor of the preestablished social structure rather than an active process in the *creation* of that social structure' (Rychlak, 1990: 17). Once conceived as merely a mediator, the individual's learning of that now all-important 'discourse' has to be explained, and social constructionism is forced into the old mediational models; Rychlak (1990) notes Harré's explicit acceptance of Hullian learning theory.

As noted above, Searle (1995) has neatly turned the question of the social construction of reality around to the question of how social reality is itself construed. When one stops to think about even common terms of social theory and interaction – terms such as *society* or *culture* or *institution* – they appear far less straightforward than might at first be the case (Williams, 1976). Further, without a clear conceptualisation of such terms as the *social* it is difficult to say what one could possibly mean by the expression 'social change'; for, unless we have a clear formulation of what it is that changes, how can we determine that it has changed (Krishna, 1965)? Moreover, some theorists (Marcuse, 1964/1970, for example) doubt that there has been anything but superficial (quantitative) change over the past half-century in which the fact and impacts of change have been so loudly touted in a context where structures have not altered; in which, that is, there has been no *qualitative* change. Thus, when we too casually refer to the realm of 'the social', and then as a determining influence on our psychological functioning, we might as equally be puzzled by the way we construct social reality as the way it constructs us.

Now, these observations of Rychlak (1990, 1993) and Searle (1995) call to mind again one conclusion from the debate between the Marxists and the existentialists, more particularly a little-known thinker who was a precursor of existentialist thinking generally, as well as the thought of Nietzsche particularly. This was Max Stirner (1845/1963) whose book *The Ego and His Own* has been characterised as one of the most impressive attacks on authoritarianism ever written. Stirner argued the case for individual freedom, freedom as self-liberation from all and any individual person, institution and, importantly here, idea or ideology that attempted to make us its slave. His clash with Marx has been argued to have generated the 'shift' in Marx's thinking from its moral (the so-called 'young Marx') to its so-called 'scientific' analysis (the 'mature Marx').

Whatever the merits of Stirner's position, and of Marx's response to it in the work which evidences the shift (*The German Ideology*), an appraisal of their debate finds an interesting conclusion to be defensible. This is that their different perspectives can be seen as two different searchlights illuminating the same territory, yet rarely intersecting (Carroll, 1974). Carroll draws attention specifically to Nietszche's viewpoint here, that 'the germs of life from which the two philosophies grow are different' (1974: 131), adding that Nietszche's work led him to doubt that a total, systematic social theory was either insightful or useful.

Thus, Rychlak's (1993) principle of complementarity has an echo in an earlier debate in social philosophy, a debate that can indeed be scored as a 'draw'. Thus, too, 'when we all recognise that although we are participants in the same endeavour, we are relying on complementary groundings for the knowledge we seek. One person's explanatory gain is therefore not the other's loss' (Rychlak, 1993: 941).

Interestingly, however, while personal construct psychology is conciliatory toward social constructionism, the reverse appears to be less the case. Indeed, social constructionism seems driven to critique and dismiss personal construct psychology in a fashion which again echoes the earlier debate in social philosophy.

From Rychlak's point of view, the 'searchlight analogy' is more appropriate, encouraging as it does a complementarity. If this is found to be unacceptable, then it would be interesting to inquire as to which perspective best accounts for the drive to abolish one perspective in favour of the other. That the social seems driven to annihilate the personal revives the older debate already noted and, moreover, perhaps directs us to the underlying personal dynamics of what Popper (1945) identified as *methodological essentialism*. This approach searches for the 'one true perspective', that is, for a single principle that reduces the complexity of life to a simple formula, such as the nature or destiny of one's race, caste, religion or class. It is, for Popper, one underpinning of an absolutist outlook he called *historicism* that characterised alike Plato, Hegel and Marx. In each of these thinkers the individual is seen as being caught up in something that is beyond individual, even perhaps human, capacity to influence. Thus, attraction to a particular style or level of analysis is related to a particular outlook on the world, one which too easily results in an authoritarianism in which 'possession of truth justifies suppression of falsehood'. The example of Weber's family life (Mitzman, 1969) and Vaihinger's disability (Vaihinger, 1911/1952) are in mind here. Put less cryptically, the attraction to a particular way of construing the world in this or that social or psychological theory might be itself influenced by other features of a construct system (Weber's troubles with his father, Vaihinger's poor eyesight); personal construct psychology is uniquely placed to illuminate these matters.

To return to the main theme here, Chiari and Nuzzo (1996a, 1996b), recognising the plethora of constructionist positions in psychology, seek to differentiate personal construct psychology from other constructionisms within psychology. They catalogue the wide variety of expressions drawn from different theorists sampled above, and suggest that the significance of other constructionisms and constructivisms for personal construct psychology is that they present cues for further useful elaboration of personal construct psychology.

Now, Chiari and Nuzzo (1996b) note a number of problems in attempting to clarify the different constructivisms. In particular, there is the problem of selecting the dimension on which such differentiation is attempted. From a number of possibilities, they suggest that the key dimension for differentiating among the various constructivist positions is the one which sees them approaching differently the knowledge–reality relationship.

Chiari and Nuzzo (1996b) suggest the label *psychological constructivism* be used only for those positions that emphasise the overcoming of the traditional realist–idealist debate that is central in considerations of the knowledge–reality relationship. Under this label, they distinguish *epistemological constructivism*, which stresses the 'ordering and organisation of a world constituted by the person's experience', and *hermeneutic constructivism*, in which 'operations of distinctions in language constitute the generation and validation of all reality' (1996b: 178). They rule out and into a different metatheory (critical or limited realist metatheory) those positions that claim 'the subjective representation of an observer-independent, "out there" reality' (1996b: 178). Thus, if personal construct psychology is understood as a realist position, it is not a psychological constructivism. However, for them it is an epistemological constructivism usefully understood in terms of a general psychological constructivism that can be elaborated by reference to both the social constructionists and the biological position of Maturana and Varela. In emphasising the epistemological aspect they echo Mancini and Semerari's (1988) account which relates the position taken by personal construct psychology to the type of shift made by Popper in epistemology proper. That is, the greater significance is given in both to the 'inner outlook' in framing our understandings of the world in terms of what we bring to our observations, in one way or another.

Chiari and Nuzzo's is a close account offered to facilitate the conversation about constructivist ideas. In like vein, a number of points might be made in response to it. First, we might recall the narrower characterisation of personal construct psychology as *gnosiology*. That is, the interest was in the constructs the person employs in interpreting the world. This was a *psychological* not an *epistemological* project, and in fact might suggest a closer connection to Chiari and Nuzzo's *hermeneutic constructivism* without going outside personal construct psychology to other positions; though this is not to say that an elaboration through the insights of social constructionists, narratological and 'biological' thinking is not valuable.

A second, and related, point is that despite Kelly's (1955/1991) observations concerning realism, it is possible to give a coherent account of personal construct psychology as consistent with a realist position; for example, in

Noaparast's (1995) terms, or in Stevens' (1998) accounts of a minimal realism, or perhaps even in Anderson's (1962) terms. Further, this need not negate hermeneutics entirely. For example, hermeneutics, when taken out of the realm of the ethereal and into the domain of lived social practice, as Habermas, for example, entreats us to do, finds us working in a real world of things; things about which we discourse, and discourse in a fashion which assumes there are real 'things' to discourse about. While the relation between personal construct psychology and hermeneutics will be later developed, it is clear from the 'realist tone' of much of Kelly's writing that the affinity with hermeneutics very much involves a notion of practice and action in and on a real world. It would appear to be the pragmatists who best elaborated the relation between our meaning-making and practical life, Dewey, in particular. Thus, the familiarity between phenomenology and pragmatism. To move too far from an influential 'real world' appears to move us away from what personal construct psychology was centrally about.

Finally, these last points are tied down from another direction in Butt's (1996) argument concerning personal construct psychology as a theory of social action, and its links to the existential tradition (Warren, 1985; Butt, 1997, 1998a, 1998b) noted previously. This shifts it away from the cognitive focus that might too tightly tie it to epistemology 'writ large', and to a relativism arising from a rejection of realism. That is, if we start with a different dimension of differentiation to one centred in epistemology, a different direction emerges for the elaboration of personal construct psychology in response to the complementary ideas arising in such perspectives as the narratological approach, and the challenges from social constructionism.

Such an approach, it might be suggested, leads equally to hermeneutics. Moreover, this is especially so when personal construct psychology is considered in terms of its origins in the psychology of pragmatism, and we note the significance for later hermeneutics of the world of practice and action. Moreover, it might be suggested that even if the realism–idealism tension is overcome in phenomenology, this will leave scope still for a *psychology*. Personal construct psychology appears to be well placed to be such a psychology. Chiari and Nuzzo (1996a: 27) emphasise that personal construct psychology is not only the first constructivist theory but the only constructivist theory of personality *and* psychotherapy. Indeed, this is worth stressing further and for two reasons. First, it reinforces Mair's (1970a) observation concerning personal construct psychology being a *psychology for* psychotherapy. Second, it draws attention to the general absence of such a focus in many other positions. In respect to social constructionism in particular, it is not clear just what psychotherapeutic consequences flow from the adoption of such a position.

Concluding comment

Personal construct psychology was developed as a psychology of the individual, an idiographic psychology. However, it nonetheless saw that individual inextricably linked to others who must be construed in one way or another; indeed, one early construction of personal construct psychology saw it as 'applying mainly to the social realm as shown by the emphasis on interpersonal constructs, roles and role playing' (Jones, 1971: 282).

The failure of critics to attend to the social dimensions of personal construct psychology, coupled with an understanding of it as merely an 'individualistic theory', and also as overly focused on cognitive matters, leads into significant conflict with social constructionist positions. The difficulties generated by these conflicts parallel a failure to attend to its realist dimension, leading into significant misidentification of it as a relativist position. Equally, the focus on epistemology may distract attention from its focus on the individual's lived-experience in a world which has to be dealt with.

Three strategies present themselves in respect to this conflict. One is to show the shortcomings of the social constructionist position which is most vigorous in its criticism of personal construct psychology; especially extremes of such position which overemphasise social influences. We could not hope to do this in any thoroughgoing way here, but have indicated the directions such a critique would take. It is a direction which critiques the implicit idealism in such a position, that is, 'the social' is taken as something analogous to the way other idealist positions take God, or Mind, or the Forms as having some higher level of operation or action in a world in which there is, rather, but one way of being. It is a direction which might also take us back to a voluminous critical literature on Marxism.

The second strategy is to suggest that social constructionism leaves too little place for individual agency, and that this must be given greater role. More of this later in Chapter 5. Related to the sentiment being expressed here, however, are the echoes of other debates that illuminate the issues; in particular the concerns of the early anarchist thinkers and later existentialists who, equally as strongly as did others, attacked the 'bourgeois' conception of the individual without losing the concept of the individual altogether.

A third strategy is to accept the opportunity for elaboration of personal construct psychology accorded by the appearance of so many constructionist and constructivist perspectives. This was the approach taken by Chiari and Nuzzo (1996a, 1996b), who also point us toward hermeneutics. In the spirit of their inquiries, the general theoretical ferment in respect of these matters sampled in this chapter is taken to assist the elaboration of personal construct psychology. However, we might not quite yet give up on personal construct psychology as already accommodating many of the insights of recent thinking and in a more comprehensive way, *vis-à-vis* psychology as a wider field of inquiry.

4   Structuralism and beyond

It is difficult to accurately assess what is on the face of it a shift or rift in the enterprise that is philosophy from about the middle of this century. Whether that shift is judged to be a superficial one, or a more fundamental one, turns around one's views as to what constitutes the endeavour that is philosophy itself. In one sense, the same problems as fascinated the ancient Greeks remain before us; there may be no new problems in philosophy, merely more urgent or pressing ones. Equally, if philosophy is concerned with the assessment of arguments and the attempt to build on established truth (Scruton, 1994), then many of the thinkers generating the shift – be it superficial or momentous – are not doing philosophy as such, and therefore might be held to touch its enterprise but little. Finally, if the project that is philosophy as conceived in 'modern' terms has not been completed, as Habermas (1981/1985) has force-fully and consistently argued, then these developments would again be relegated to a less significant place for philosophy. Thereby, we might 'learn from the mistakes of those extravagant programs which have tried to negate modernity' rather than give up modernity and its project as a lost cause (Habermas, 1981/1985: 12).

On the other hand, if the exercise that is philosophy rests on the notion of a reflective self seeking real knowledge of the world, then recent developments are a problem for that very exercise. The argument that that self is from the moment of the commencement of gazing at the world already gazing in a certain way undercuts this notion. Thus, if philosophy implies an activity of a 'subject', an individual perceiving, thinking, making determinations about things in the world, and so forth, then there is a problem emerging from an argument that from the very beginning that subject is already embedded in a discourse that constrains both the questions and answers of traditional philosophy.

Thus, the shift in philosophy may be evaluated, particularly with the type of hindsight that we now use in looking backwards to the birth of 'modern' philosophy, as being as significant as that change brought by Kant. Kant's enterprise began the move of philosophy from its ancient roots to a more modern, less metaphysical philosophy that Hegel was to complete (Redding, 1996). Thus, the developments recognised as structuralism, poststructuralism and postmodernity may, on the one hand, be dismissed as mere restatements of scepticism and as saying nothing particularly challenging for philosophy – whatever their own problems in terms of comprehensibility – or, alternatively, accepted as casting the very enterprise of philosophy in a new light, perhaps even as being an impossible enterprise. While the jury is still out on the matter and may be for some time, a judgement along the lines of these developments at minimum overstating their case may well emerge (Searle, 1995; Sokal and Bricmont, 1997), even though some degree or level of crisis might be identified for philosophy as a discipline (Cohen and Dascal, 1989/1991), and some degree of compromise felt to be needed and available (Frank, 1984/1989).

Passmore, in his effort to augment his earlier *A Hundred Years of Philosophy*, despairs of being able to describe briefly a field that had become chaotic, 'ill-defined, immensely variegated in aspiration and method . . . [with] . . . [s]o many philosophers writing, so many problems raised' (1985: 1). Almost a decade later, Scruton (1994), in a survey of modern philosophy, distinguishes *modern* from *modernist*. For him, English-speaking philosophy was modern but not modernist, while recent French philosophy (the chief exponents of which he identified as Foucault and Derrida) was modernist rather than modern. The distinction turned around whether a philosophy based itself on the assessment of arguments and the desire to build on previously established truths (modern), or seeks to find truths that are novel and discontinuous with the past (modernist). So distrustful of the past is the modernist, according to Scruton, that he or she seeks to be ahead of the times; hence, 'post-modern'.

It is difficult to read these last types of critical survey, and the works to which they refer, without concluding that something happened in and to philosophy around the late 1950s and early 1960s; though specific dates are always challengeable (Foster, 1985). As noted, several developments are implicated in this as far as philosophy is concerned, chiefly a rediscovery of the significance of language, and the extension of the insights of linguistics and of the sociology of knowledge into philosophy. All together, these developments moved to centre stage some key concepts that took on the mantle of 'movements' in thought: structuralism, its 'completion' in poststructuralism, perhaps a neo-structuralism (Frank, 1984/1989), and postmodernism as a more embracing term for poststructuralism and sometimes postrational perspectives.

Kelly (1955/1991) is unlikely to have been too familiar with the controversies brewing in Europe in the late 1950s that were to reach English-speaking readers around the time his own major work was going to press and being reviewed. Nonetheless, in the present context it is of value to test the alignment of personal construct psychology with these developments because they feed into contemporary debates which personal construct psychology cannot easily ignore.

This test or assessment of personal construct psychology against these controversies and developments is, though, a difficult task, and for various reasons. First, these 'isms' themselves are not clear-cut or as coherent as bodies of interrelated ideas in the way that, say, Marxism or fascism might be taken to be; even though Marxism and fascism have their own internal differences and tensions. Second, in some cases what is observed is one or a few basic ideas in one field, being 'applied' or finding their way into other fields; thereby posing a problem of hybridisation and possibly being as distracting as they are challenging in the new field. Finally, the developments themselves did not stagnate; rather, sometimes by reason of their own inner logics, they were overtaken; structuralism by poststructuralism, for example. Given the complexity of these matters and the continuing debate around them, it is a intimidating task to attempt an evaluation. Fortunately, however, what is primarily required here is a critical outline rather than a critique.

Structuralism and poststructuralism

As Sturrock (1986) indicates, structuralism arose from a confluence of ideas already influential in Western Europe in the 1960s. A more specific origin, however, is usually located in developments following on from the ideas of the Swiss linguist Ferdinand de Saussure (1857–1913), who took up the definition of structure as 'an autonomous entity of internal dependencies' (Lavers, 1982). These developments found those ideas that had originated in linguistics emerging in social science, particularly in the work of Lévi-Strauss (1958/1963), who was self-consciously a structuralist. These same ideas were given a more specifically political focus through the particular approach to literary criticism demanded by Roland Barthes (1964/1967, 1957/1973). In relation to psychology, while Gestalt psychology is already implicated with phenomenology as a major tributary in the development of structuralism, Foucault and Lacan provide structuralist perspectives in psychology, focused particularly on psychoanalysis. What the confluence of ideas produced in all of these fields – and however comfortable the individual thinkers just identified with the term might be – was essentially a *methodology* (Sturrock, 1979, 1986).

The methodology that was, or is, structuralism approaches the various disciplines with the question of what underlies the 'givens' of any situation addressed by that discipline. That is, the method is to look for a deeper level of truth or reality beneath what is immediately obvious in a particular domain; it was significantly a critical mode of thought as earlier characterised in philosophy. In language, where it had its origin, the method pointed to a superficial level of the 'sign' which was underpinned by a level of the 'signifier'. Thus the thing to which the sign, say, 'cigar' is applied is obvious, but the wealth and power signified by cigar smoking lies beneath that obvious level as telling a great deal more about a situation in which a simple statement like 'he was smoking a cigar' is made. In psychology, Turkle (1978) draws attention to Lacan's interest in Freud's 'Rat-Man' case, which is equally illustrative of the sign/symbol distinction, and the teasing out of the symbolic connections. The

Rat-Man's 'presenting problem', as we might now say, concerned anxieties and dreams of being attacked by rats (*Ratten*); however, there were uncovered significant conflicts in his life turning around his disappointment in his father who had died leaving gambling debts which the son had to pay off by instalments (*Raten*). Further, he had some unresolved grief and other feelings concerning the death in infancy of his sister (Rita), and he was experiencing a deal of uncertainty as to whether he should go through with a marriage (*hieratten*) (Turkle, 1978: 252).

It is interesting to note that Lévi-Strauss (1958/1963) was very much concerned to avoid relativism. He was concerned to discover or illuminate fundamental social and mental processes that the different social and cultural institutions had arisen to express. In a reply to some of his critics, he objects to any relativistic notions that might be assumed from his studies, in particular to a 'static relativism' that leads to a blind support for the status quo of the researcher's own society, or, on the other hand, the repudiation of the idea of 'progress'. As he notes: 'I denounce it [static relativism] as a danger ever present in the anthropologists path' and, he rather expresses two 'apparently contradictory attitudes, namely, respect for societies very different from our own, and active participation in the transformation of our own' (1963: 335).

Of course, before this methodology took on its specific meaning, there was in Marx a similar methodology in the manner in which a particular structuring principle, that is, social class, determined a whole range of things at the level of culture and consciousness. This was formally expressed in the central tenet of Marxism, *historical materialism*. That is, the so-called economic base, which described the manner in which human beings organise themselves to work and produce, *determines* the form and content of the law, morality, attitudes in art and education, modes of consciousness, and so on, at the level of the 'superstructure'. Indeed, Marxism always remained a strong influence on structuralist thought, though whether, as Scruton asserts, 'the "general science of signs" promised by Saussure lent itself to [the] radical political agenda' and provided a 'method for "decoding" the artefacts and conventions of bourgeois society, so as to expose their meaning' (1994: 268) is beyond our interests to explore. Scruton's observations do, however, expose the intensity of reactions to that 'peculiar aberration called "structuralist criticism", whose pseudo-scientific jargon and radical message is taken one stage further by its successor – the "deconstructionist criticism" of Derrida' (Scruton, 1994: 268).

In summary, across the different thinkers identified as structuralist, what is privileged is the signifier rather than the signified:

> The same signifier is sure to have different signifieds for two different people, occupying a differently defined semantic space because of the dissimilarity of individual experience; again, the same signifier will have different signifieds for the same person at different times, since configuration of our semantic space is never stable. Structuralism invites us to

delight in the plurality of meaning this opens up, to reject the authoritarian or unequivocal interpretation of signs.

(Sturrock, 1979: 15)

That these developments occurred in France is an interesting observation in the history and sociology of ideas, though in allowing such origins the work of the North American philosopher C.S. Peirce (1829–1914) is too easily overlooked. Indeed, Colapietro (1990) has forcefully argued in the context of that 'decentring of the subject' that resulted from the developments in French intellectual life that the American pragmatists had already taken us further and without the same loss of the subject as *agent*.

Poststructuralism is 'post' in the sense of following on from, rather than rejecting, the fundamental position. Derrida (1967/1973, 1967/1976) is the most radical of the theorists who wish to reject 'structure' for 'structuring', that is, that the influences acting on the individual, the context in which the individual is inescapably immersed, represent a series of chaotic 'environments'. Derrida finds western philosophy working with notions of logic and language that are taken to be transcendental of experience rather than immanent within it and thus as relative as is all else. Structuralism, he argues, smuggles in a form of idealism by seeing language as 'revealing of' rather than creating meaning (Sturrock, 1986), and Derrida's deconstruction is an attempt to expose this error along with the dominance of certain logical principles which have been taken as fixed laws of thought, but which are in fact merely relative themselves.

With a spectrum of opinion ranging from the view that Derrida merely inflated the significance and impact of the simple idea of an extreme pluralism of viewpoints in society, to a dismissal of his work as merely a composite of assertions, it is difficult to assess the type of position he represents. We might not wish to accept Searle's assessment, 'What is one to do . . . in the face of an array of weak or even nonexistent arguments for a conclusion that seems preposterous?' (1995: 160), but in moving too much further there is the very real problem of facing a much bigger task than is appropriate here. Moreover, matters moved on and poststructuralism is best considered as part of postmodernism with which it is reasonably taken as synonymous.

More recently, Frank (1984/1989) has reexamined the development of the ideas deriving from structuralism and assessed their contemporary significance. Frank's argument seeks a middle way between French poststructuralism and German hermeneutics. He develops a position that tries to preserve the insights of both modern and postmodern thinking. More specifically, he attempts to square the idea of human dignity and individual autonomy with the fact of the construction of the individual by linguistic, cultural and historical orderings of those same individuals.

Structuralism, then, had either significant or overrated implications for philosophy, depending on the position one took in respect of both structuralism and philosophy. There is in fact yet another interesting parallel here with the philosophical implications and impacts of -ism. Marx himself left the field of philosophy in disgust with a stinging criticism in his 'The Holy Family' (1844b), a criticism he found it necessary to repeat in 'The German Ideology' written in 1845–6 though unpublished in full until 1932. In these works, he relegated philosophy to the domain of empty criticism, which he summed up in his 'Eleventh Thesis on Feuerbach' (1845): 'The Philosophers have only *interpreted* the world in various ways; the point is to *change* it.' Philosophy, as an exercise in understanding the world, was to give way to advocacy of a better way of life (the 'classless society') and agitation for change.

If structuralism is accorded philosophical significance, this judgement derives from the claim that it calls for a significant change in the way philosophy is done or conceives of its task. Yet, as both Passmore (1985) and Scruton (1994) have suggested, there are major difficulties with the ideas of the thinkers identified above. Their positions leave many unresolved questions and issues and they focus on a level of human activity that is at one remove from that focused on by traditional philosophy. Nonetheless, these ideas set in motion forces that were to grow in strength.

Modernity and postmodernity

In an interesting 'twist' Baum (1988) identified Darwin, Marx and Freud as 'doctors of modernity', yet found their impact in terms of their *irrationality* and their denigration of the creative power of the human mind, a charge that is more often brought against postmodernity. Such are the complexities of identification and delineation of thought in the contemporary intellectual scene. Equally illustrative of this complexity is the collection of thinkers identified with the term postmodern, and the *differences* between their accounts; more so when those accounts themselves display change and sometimes reversals over time. Foucault (1982) is a case in point in respect of the latter claim, suggesting very late in his career that he might have underestimated the importance of the individual and overestimated the deadening impact of the themes of the Enlightenment.

Postmodernity, is, again, an extension of modernity in the manner of the relationship suggested of structuralism and poststructuralism. That said, the terms postmodernism, postmodernity and postmodernist all defy definition. Lyotard does attempt a definition of postmodernism: 'I define *postmodern* as incredulity toward metanarratives' (1979/1984: xxiv). Metanarratives are 'grand narratives', stories that go to legitimise particular practices, like, for example, science. The *modern* is particularly implicated in the use of metanarratives and Lyotard suggests examples of these: 'the dialectics of Spirit, the hermeneutics of meaning, the emancipation of the rational or working subject, the creation of wealth' (1979/1984: xxiii).

Lyotard elaborates the postmodern in terms of a situation in which the old metanarratives are dispersed in 'clouds of narrative language elements', of which the individual inhabits or is immersed in at any one time. The image is, on the one hand, that of rupture and discontinuity with all of the past grand explanations. On the other hand, there is an image of infinite variety in the present, a variety of inconsistent expectations that are only apparently managed by applying a logic that derives from what is a most chaotic level of practice, that is, the logic of technology. An illusion of a determinable system – not the reality of local or regional determinism by reason of the incommensurability of the mixtures of language clouds in which we are immersed – is maintained by allocating 'our lives for the growth of power' (1979/1984: xxiv). Across the whole of life in advanced technological society, 'the legitimation of that power is based on its optimising the system's performance – efficiency' (1979/1984: xxiv). It becomes an obvious truth that the principle of efficient performance is to be applied even as we understand and experience its inconsistencies. Our own incredulity, however, has grown to a point that we no longer anticipate any hope of significant change.

Now, Lyotard's account of the postmodern is challenging material that has wedded the type of critique of life governed by advanced technology that the philosophers of technology had been mounting to suggestions about language and the grand accounts of the human condition. While those last accounts had sustained people and provided security, they are also exposed as restrictive and serving of particular, as opposed to general, interests. Thus, postmodernism represents a suspension of belief in all of the grand stories of the past, and a similar outlook in respect to the motifs of the present; in short, discontinuity and an absence of a grounding for our knowledge and belief, beyond local discourses which sustain particular, local knowledge and belief.

Now, as is the way of things, these views do not go unchallenged and at least a note of some lines of challenge is appropriate here. At the outset, however, we might recall the tradition from Vico to Vaihinger earlier discussed. What those thinkers were emphasising was the importance of 'grand narratives', 'fictions', 'myths', and the like; the importance not of any particular myths, but of myth-making. To suggest that humankind might dispose of myth-making might appear rather radical surgery for the problem that particular myths operating in the contemporary scene are identified as subjugating. Indeed, the rejection of grand narratives may too easily itself take on the aura of a grand narrative, a 'common wisdom'.

Norris (1992) argued against all of the 'posts' and 'neos' in terms of the loss of historical understanding and the *total* dismissal of Enlightenment values. He (Norris, 1993) responded to critics and developed his theme more forcefully; that is, in essence, that postmodern theoretical insights are rather more shallow than they are deep. Moreover, a too ready rejection of the usefulness of such notions as truth, reason, critique, ideology and false consciousness by postmodern thinkers stampedes us into an uncritical acceptance of popular opinion. The too easy acceptance of a closed, authoritarian outlook would be one disturbing consequence of this, an outlook that rules out all but a 'sanctioned' wisdom about how the world is.

These views continue a debate that has found postmodernism construed as both a postmodernism of reaction and a postmodernism of resistance (Foster, 1985). The first provides in the end but a strengthening of the status quo by seeing debates over even radically differing alternatives as still debates about 'style', still debates within culture conceived as 'neutral' or 'benign'. The second, a postmodernism of resistance, rather constitutes a 'counter-practice ... concerned with a critical deconstruction of tradition', a questioning rather than an acceptance of concealed social and political affili-ations with a 'benign' culture (Foster, 1985: xii).

The point here, then, is that we may have been bedazzled by the scope of the claims of postmodernism. Worse, we may have been lulled into a compla-cency that makes us easy targets for whatever fad or fashion is invented to amuse us. Dostoevsky's concerns for the quality of life under conditions of advanced technology, the power of which attracted a developing fascination in his time, are prophetic for the type of concerns gaining strength in response to a rampant postmodernism:

> The Crystal Palace is Dostoevsky's crowning symbol for the barrenness of industrial civilization [where] everything will be provided, man's every desire will be satisfied. He will be insulated from pain – but the more he becomes the automaton consumer the more he will also suffer from excruciating boredom ... become imaginatively imbecilic. Boredom will drive him to acts of the most vicious, gratuitous cruelty and sadism.
>
> (Carroll, 1974: 149)

Psychology and postmodernity

When one turns specifically to the discipline that is psychology, we are fortu-nate that there have been other labourers in the field in respect to its relations to postmodernism. Kvale (1992), for example, provides a valuable and, impor-tantly, critical review of the possible impact of postmodernism on psychology, and also usefully summarises the material being sampled above. He notes three senses of the expression *postmodern*: first, *postmodernity*, referring to the postmodern age; second, *postmodernism*, referring to the cultural expres-sions of that age; and, third, *postmodern thought*, referring to philosophical reflection on both the age and the culture (Kvale, 1992: 2).

The first is characterised by the loss of certain ideas arising with the Enlightenment; that is, the naive belief in release from inner and outer oppres-sion, and progress through research and the growth of knowledge. Significantly, this brings a loss of the concept of an objective reality. The second is represented by a kaleidoscope of expression through the various forms of media, a form and content that leaves one in significant doubt about there being any distinction between reality and fantasy. The third, more inter-esting for present purposes, is that collapsing of observer and observed, the constructed nature of reality (through language) as against its 'givenness', the rejection of the notion that there are 'foundations' of knowledge, and, of course, the loss of the individual, the 'decentring' of the subject.

Now, what would psychology look like when 'done' in a postmodernist way or as an example of postmodern thought? One answer is that psychology as it has become would be significantly critiqued, and the very possibility of a postmodern psychology questioned; such would be seen as 'a contradiction in terms' (Kvale, 1992: 31). The thrust of this argument is that psychology as the science of the subject is made redundant when the subject, that is, the notion of an isolated self or ego, is jettisoned (Gergen, 1985, 1991). Alternatively, psychology might move 'out of the archaeology of the psyche and into the cultural landscape of the present world, directly entering a postmodern discourse' (Kvale, 1992: 53)

This last possibility is urged by Gergen (1992). After reviewing the apparently quite devastating impact of postmodern thought for psychology, he offers a number of possibilities for the way in which 'postmodern thought opens vistas of untold significance for the discipline' of psychology (1992: 25). Chiefly, these are: technological advance, cultural critique and the construction of new worlds.

The first is a recognition that such things as testing for psychological deficits, skills training, development of therapeutic methods, sensitivity training to minority-group needs and interests, and so forth, would remain appropriate. Here, however, the technologies of effective intervention ('knowing how') are separated from any truth claims that might be made about the descriptions and explanations that are offered for them; that is, any 'knowing that' aspects. In short, as long as terms like 'deficit' or 'performance' are not objectified but 'remain sensitive and open to the social and evaluational implications . . . then such technologies would be congenial with postmodernism' (Gergen, 1992: 26).

The second flows from the first and is premised on the sensitive relationship between these technologies and human life. Thus a postmodern psychology is to serve as a device for maintaining what we might call a role of 'eternal vigilance' over the mystifying and objectifying tendencies in life governed by advanced technology. The psychologist is to discard an assumed value-neutral position and join together 'the personal, the professional and the political' (Gergen, 1992: 27) as a way of consciously remaining within a context, yet serving the purpose of emancipation from the mystifications attempted to be perpetuated by that context.

The third is an invitation to 'conjecture boldly', to contribute to cultural change through generating new ways of thinking. The psychologist of the postmodern era is to be a scholar 'willing to be audacious, to break barriers of common sense by offering new forms of theory, of interpretation, of intelligibility' (Gergen, 1992: 27).

Gergen's (1985, 1991, 1992) is but one voice among many which articulates the challenges and the possible responses for psychology as a discipline faced with the postmodern culture and forms of postmodern thought. Other voices are raised within the same volume to which his last observations contributed. However, there are different responses, even to his own analysis. In that same volume in which Gergen outlined the directions for a postmodern psychology, Chaiklin (1992) offered a different view of postmodern psychology. Further, Mascolo and Dalto (1995) and Botella (1995) have fixed our critical attention on postmodernism from a constructionist perspective, specifically in relation to personal construct psychology.

Chaiklin (1992) argues that postmodern philosophy is not easily assimilated to psychological questions, perhaps raising as many problems as it resolves. Further, he echoes an earlier observation that the concepts of 'postmodern' and 'modern' in respect of psychology are not at all clear. Finally, he argues that there are other ways forward in respect of accommodating the types of concerns raised for psychology by postmodern thought, in particular, cultural-historical psychology that does not draw its theoretical sustenance from postmodernism. He concludes that in the attempts to show the relevance of postmodern psychology for psychology that he has reviewed, not much is offered by postmodern thought for the goals of psychology, or even for the goals postmodernist thinkers themselves put forward for psychology.

From a different direction, Kendall and Michael (1997) argue, and Michael and Kendall (1997) defend, the assessment that postmodern social psychology is less innovative and rather a 'much more "mundane" activity than its protagonists would like to think' (Kendall and Michael, 1997: 8). The work of Gergen (1991, 1992) is significantly centred in their argument and Gergen (1997) replies in usual forceful fashion, reiterating his position that privileges social processes over the individual in terms of the origination of whatever phenomenon is under consideration in social psychology.

Mascolo and Dalto (1995) propose a critique of Gergen (1991) from within a constructionist framework, a critique that has particular significance to personal construct psychology. Their thesis is that the image of the 'saturated self' Gergen has sketched represents an overstatement and that there is a need to retain a place for human *agency* in constructionist models of human functioning. They outline a number of directions for allowing *both* the social and the personal-agency dimension to be accorded due weight. One important dimension suggested is the work of socio-cultural psychologists, a suggestion that parallels Chaiklin's (1992) challenge that all that is in postmodern psychology is already accommodated within cultural-historical psychology.

Botella (1995) offers a most clearsighted and helpful paper for the present theme. He addresses the issue of personal construct psychology in relation to postmodernism, reiterating our earlier concerns in noting the vexing preliminary problem that any alignment of personal construct psychology with postmodern thought has to first determine just what constitutes the latter. He reminds us that there are wider and more restricted understandings of postmodernism, and indicates that a different alignment will be observed depending on which understanding of the term we have. At the most extreme, postmodernism is understood as descriptive of a situation of total relativism in which there is no means of evaluating one world-view against another in a context of many world-views, and where reality and fiction are blurred. A more formal understanding, however, drawing on Polkinghorne (1992), sees it as a reaction to the optimism of the modernist project in epistemology, but not leading to the extreme form of relativism just noted; rather it leads back to a form of pragmatism in epistemology. Thus are given four basic themes of a positive understanding of postmodern epistemology: foundationlessness, fragmentation, constructivism and neo-pragmatism (Polkinghorne, 1992). The last theme saves us from total relativism in epistemology by providing criteria, albeit 'local criteria', for making judgements; essentially the abductive method noted earlier. In this respect, the 'neo-pragmatism' that is being referred to is in the psychological tradition of Dewey and James, rather than the philosophical focus of Peirce, as discussed in Chapter 2.

On this understanding of postmodern thought, Botella (1995) finds personal construct psychology harmonised with that thought to a significant degree but with some refined distinctions. Thus, it is compatible with an acceptance that we cannot access 'reality' directly, but must deal with it through our constructions of it (foundationlessness), with pragmatism, and obviously with construction. However, the theme of fragmentariness needs to be examined more carefully. Fragmentariness as emphasising the significance of 'the local and situated, instead of the general and totalizing' (Botella, 1995: 21), needs to be considered differently for the *content* of construing and for the *process* of construing.

The content of construing will be idiosyncratic and contribute to an idiographic psychology. However, the process of construing is something that is shared, and understanding of shared construing can contribute to a nomothetic understanding in psychology. Thus might personal construct psychology avoid that relativism that has been the chief dilemma of postmodern thought. Personal construct psychology is not a relativistic psychology, not an acceptance of 'anything goes'. Rather, it held from the start that constructions are 'tested', not just held on to in the face of everything. Indeed, Botella echoes the familiar criticism of relativism in his discussion, noting, however, that other forms of constructivism are also often mistakenly characterised as relativistic. Thus Maturana and Varella (1984/1987) posit a process of avoiding dogma and solipsism alike; and narrative psychology in some forms at least posits 'better' meanings in terms of the scope and range of stories, and their subsumption of narrower themes of a life.

Solas (1995) provides a similar discussion to Botella (1995) in respect of an extreme form of postmodern thought in deconstruction. Focusing on the social aspects of personal construct psychology, he draws out similarities and differences between the position of Derrida and personal construct psychology. The general similarity lies in the significance each gives to the manner in which our constructions are intimately connected to those of others in both a validating and an invalidating fashion, as well as in terms of shared, but not identical, meanings. The difference, stressed also by Mair

(1989), lies in the degree of emphasis on language and its relation to thought accepted by each perspective. For deconstruction, language is the essential element of thought; for personal construct psychology, there is or appears to be an idea of language existing in a kind of 'storage space' unconnected to forms of discourse (Leman, 1970).

Solas (1995), however, considers deconstruction along lines suggested by Mair (1989) for its value in extending or illuminating the personal construct psychology perspective. Each shares a view of the world as existing independently of our perceptions of it, but whereas personal construct psychology sees that world the way, we might say, a physicist might see it (Fransella, 1983), Derrida sees it as composed not only of physical properties but also of social properties consisting of institutions and institutionalised forms that have a different place in respect to our construing of the world than do its physical properties. These institutional forms have to be seen as not just features to be construed but as causal, originating sources of construing itself. This begs some questions of course, questions concerning the construction of social reality (Searle, 1995), but these are not presently relevant.

In general terms and most simply put, personal construct psychology is a psychology that is touched only marginally by these developments and when they have something useful to say that is arguably already significantly accommodated within personal construct psychology itself. This last is particularly the case with regard to the commonality and sociality corollaries, but not only in that respect. Personal construct psychology is relatively silent on the origins of personal constructs and, as suggested elsewhere (Warren, 1985), may well constitute a *psychology* for earlier macro-level accounts of the human condition such as that offered by Marxism. Thus, too, it appears to offer, if chiefly by default, a congenial psychology for contemporary accounts that focus on the same macro-level.

An example of the location of personal construct psychology in terms of these developments can usefully be given by reference to the earlier example of the significance of the word 'cigar'. While 'cigar' may well signify social class and power in capitalist society, or nothing whatsoever to, say, a Highlander in New Guinea – thereby meaning something by meaning nothing (Rowe, 1978) – it will signify a wide range of things to different individuals. For example, to a child who observes his father smoking a cigar it might mean that father is in a 'good mood' and tonight I will not be beaten, or that father has had a win at the casino and I might expect some small treat, or that he has been with his influential mates and will have grandiose schemes to try out on mum and there will follow argument and distress for us all. Whether cigars do or do not have a general, social significance will be of less concern to the child in this example that what it means personally to him or her.

It is not our task here to try to 'save' psychology from postmodernism, but one comment is worth making – aside from other reservations about the deeper integrity of the assertions and 'facts' of postmodern culture as derived through postmodernist thought. This is that psychology has been and continues to be radically reappraised outside of any criticsims levelled by postmodern thought – for example, by Lewin (1931), Rychlak (1970), Koch (1973), Sullivan (1984), Hillner (1987) – but in terms of what it has become, not what it 'essentially is'. The social philosopher Georges Sorel (1895) makes a related and illustrative point about science. He distinguishes science as it had become, that is, deformed by demands for practical solutions to problems of industry and technology and merely a puzzle-solving activity; and as it essentially was. The last was as *inquiry*, critical inquiry that was *disinterested* in the sense that the *activity* took a phenomenon under study in its own terms and wherever that inquiry led; as opposed to inquiry to serve some ulterior purpose. His examples of disinterested activity, which must be differentiated from 'uninterested' activity, were the artist, the warrior and the scientist. The values championed by disinterestedness are 'initiative, emulation, care for exactitude and rejection of the notion of "reward"' (Anderson, 1962: 187), disinterestedness characterised also as an outlook that stands out 'from the wrangle of special interests' (Anderson, 1962: 104).

Thus, perhaps, with psychology. The concept of inquiry into the 'behaving' of human beings – as differentiated from their (merely) observable 'behaviour', following Koch (1973) – is as justifiable as it was with the ancients. However, the collapse of this into narrowly empirical, positivistic, experimental science no different to that through which the natural world was to be approached is another matter. That other matter, moreover, was equally well critiqued from within psychology, already expressing thereby, perhaps, one aspect of science as critical inquiry into human behaving.

Postmodernism in psychology is, then, equally as problematic as it is more generally. However it is elaborated *vis-à-vis* psychology generally, two points suggest themselves as an outcome of reflection on postmodernism for personal construct psychology specifically. One is that personal construct psychology does not appear to be greatly impacted on. The other is that what is required of it by postmodernism is, again, a development of an existing social dimension of personal construct psychology which is reasonably easily achieved.

Concluding comment

Poststructuralism and postmodernism are developments in the history of thought that are themselves still in the process of elaboration and critical evaluation. Perhaps a best case scenario in respect of them is that they have deepened our understanding of the complexity of human existence under conditions of advanced technology, especially our understanding of the significance of language. A worst case scenario is that the significance of structural features and language is overstated, and that postmodernism in particular leads to obscurantism, the 'dead end' of relativism, and apathy and impotence in the face of forces that would reinstate authoritarian and anti-human regimes of life. In the case of the worst case scenario, personal construct psychology might simply remain non-responsive to whatever post-modern criticism was levelled at it, engaging in an insurrectionist passive resistance to assertions that are arguably incomprehensible and absurd. Equally, it might see as mundane the insights of poststructuralist thought in terms of its own ready acknowledgement of the extra-individual forces at play on the individual.

In the case of the best case scenario, it appears that personal construct psychology, properly understood, is one of the least objectionable psychologies for the type of issues to which we are being alerted by postmodernist arguments. Given the developing criticism of the excesses of postmodern thinking and the growing critical literature, a position mid-way between such thinking itself being evaluated as most insightful, on the one hand, and as obscurantist, on the other, might be sensibly adopted.

Personal construct psychology appears to be in something of a 'no lose' situation in respect of these developments. That is, if the disclosures of post-modern thinking are 'true', then what is required is a psychology that fits with those disclosures. With the exception of its alleged overemphasis of the indi-vidual, personal construct psychology appears to least offend a modest account of the basic tenets of postmodern thinking as outlined by Polkinghorne (1992) and developed specifically for personal construct psychology by, for example, Botella (1995) and Mascolo and Dalto (1995).

If a more radical message is suggested by postmodern thinking, then this has a more difficult and preliminary path to tread in establishing its own cred-ibility. Various commentators have drawn attention to its excesses (Norris, 1993; Searle, 1995; Sokal and Bricmont, 1997). Further, on a radical reading of postmodernism, psychology would appear to be redundant and our time wasted in pursuing it as a discipline.

Personal construct psychology appears to be well placed in respect of all of these developments. It is 'modern' in the sense that it is avowedly part of a tradition of thought stretching back over the centuries. Indeed, the perspec-tive of the centuries is championed against that of the 'flicker of passing moments' (Kelly, 1955/1991: I, 3/I, 3) in understanding humankind. While Kelly's debt to others is casually or most economically acknowledged there are acceptances and rejections of various thinkers and ideas, as noted in an earlier chapter, that link personal construct psychology both directly and indi-rectly to various strands of western thought. Yet, the constructive alternativism that is at the heart of personal construct psychology offers both a theory and a developed methodology that at least in part goes to the concerns of all but the most ardent advocates of postmodernity.

This said, one significant sticking point between postmodern thinking and psychology in general, and personal construct psychology in particular, is the relative significance of the individual, or of the notion of the *self*. Thus we turn specifically to these matters by way of opening up the magnitude of the issue and attempting something of a salvage operation for the endangered self.

5 The problem of the self

The notion of the self

What a trouble the idea of the individual, the self, the subject, the 'I', the ego, has been! When Marcuse (1941) noted the loss of the individual with the post-war final victory of advanced technology over human life, he drew attention to a shift in the conceptualisation of the individual. The notion of an individual as 'the subject of certain fundamental standards and values which no external authority was supposed to encroach on' (1941: 415) gave way to a new notion. This was of the individual as the recipient of a range of commodities and services – for many of which a 'false need' had been created – through which, and only through which, individuality was realised. The technological abolition of the individual was reflected in the decline of the family as a force in promoting difference, and in its place the premature, mass socialising of individuals through a 'system of extra-familial agents and agencies' meant that 'the generic atom becomes directly a social atom' (Marcuse, 1955/1969: 87).

Marcuse's was a lament for the loss of something that in other views 'never was', or never should have been, or never should have been in the particular conceptualisation that had become entrenched; that is, in the last case, a view of an autonomous, reflective centre of awareness that viewed the world with objectivity. This was the view within the liberal-rational tradition of western thought which saw the self as above all else *rational* (Carroll, 1974). A view within the competing Marxist-socialist tradition (there were other socialisms) saw the individual as *malleable*, that is, significantly – if not entirely or totally – a product of social forces. Both, however, had that individual contained under an image of *homo economicus*, a being who above all else is concerned to maximise possessions, driven by a rational acquisitiveness. A concept of self in the lesser known anarcho-psychological tradition stressed the *uniqueness* and *individuality* of the self. Celebrated here was our non-rational, passionate, sensuous nature, and enjoyment of and a complete immersion in Life was argued against the demands of the image of *homo economicus*.

In the chief exponents of this third tradition identified by Carroll (1974), that is, Stirner, Nietszche and Dostoevsky, there were three central critiques.

The rejection of the image of *homo economicus* asserted other values that were held to be closer to our real nature if we were not deluded by the two other traditions and the various abstractions they visited upon us; abstractions like Hegel's *Mind* or *Spirit* or Feuerbach's *Humanity* were examples, but equally 'truth' or 'the revolution' served the same purpose. The rejection of *ideology* was a rejection of the set of ideas from which these last abstractions issued. Finally, the insistence on an important subjective element in knowledge and knowing paved the way for this aspect of existentialism. These three critiques combined as an indictment of the dehumanising impacts of technology, reaching their most forceful statement on Dostoevsky's writing, noted earlier.

The liberal-rationalist view of the self has again come under renewed attack in recent times. Various writers have critiqued that view and proffered alternatives more consistent with the so-called postmodern thinking that has challenged intellectual life generally. Thus Foucault (1982, 1978/1988), Gergen (1991), Peters and Marshall (1993) and Marshall (1997), among many others, develop a number of ideas to argue the 'exhaustion of the philosophy of the subject and the bankruptcy of one particular set of liberal practices and institutions based on this paradigm' (Peters and Marshall, 1993: 20). Indeed, Van Reijen (1992: 311) expresses the core of the tensions between modernism and postmodernism as the tensions between the self thought of, on the one side, as autonomous, and, on the other, as heteronomous.

As has been intimated, there is a *déjà vu* of an older debate here. That debate crystallises in tensions between Marxism and existentialism; and does so even before existentialism was a specifically recognisable intellectual force. This tension was already in the shift in Marx's thinking generated significantly by the work of Stirner (1844/1963), who exposed various illusory concepts in Marx's early thinking. Stirner was the most ardent supporter of 'egoism', and the manner in which various 'causes' distract the individual from questions of his or her own individual being, leading in the worst case to *submission*. Stirner argues a most forceful case against *anything* being allowed to distract one from sovereignty over one's own life. He particularly points to 'ideas', ideas like 'truth', or 'science' or 'humanity', but in general any abstract concept that the individual is supposed to serve. Herein is a conception of the individual that was as antagonistic to the liberal conception as was historical Marxism and contemporary postmodern and postrational perspectives. Yet, it championed a view of the individual as recalcitrant, unpredictable, non-rational (even irrational), but equally refusing to submit to consumerist pressures and the slavish mentality that was maintained by what would now be called 'grand narratives'.

For Stirner, what he called the 'ego' referred to what was 'left out' when an individual was spoken of in terms of, say, being a 'person' or a 'true individual' or a member of a particular nation-state, a man or a woman. These abstractions stand for commonalities when what he was concerned with was not what one shares with others but those features which are not common. The nature of the self or ego was beyond words, indeterminate and uncapturable in a theoretical formulation. It was, however, a precondition or presupposition for any reflection or action in or on the world and something we know intimately from the 'inside'.

There is in fact a rich continuity of thought in relation to the individual, the self and the person stretching from the classical philosophers like Leibniz, Locke, Spinoza and Descartes to close metaphysical analysis (Strawson, 1959) and substantial commentary in older psychology and social psychology (for example, James, 1907a; Mead, 1948). Whatever else this continuity might suggest, it indicates that the notion of the self did not appear only nor merely in response to the social forces of capitalism.

Arguably the most insightful conceptualisation of the self was made almost a century ago by William James. James (1907a) introduced the metaphor of a 'stream of consciousness', in which numerous 'egos' might be seen to exist as 'pulses' or momentary 'congealings' in the stream. James stressed continuity and flux in what it is that is 'I', self or ego; just as Kant in his postulation of pure ego (the *subject* of knowing), empirical ego (the stream of consciousness, my awareness of my thoughts and feelings 'flitting' here and there) and noumenal ego (the subject of moral decisions and conduct) attempts to take more account of the fixed or enduring aspects.

James' position takes account of both the 'unity and diversity' of self. For James, the consciousness of self involves a stream of thought, each part of which as 'I' can (i) remember those which went before, and know the things they knew; and (ii) emphasise and care paramountly for certain ones among them as 'me', and *appropriate to these* the rest; this 'me' is an empirical aggregate of things objectively known. The *I* which knows them cannot itself be an aggregate, neither for psychological purposes need it be considered to be an unchanging metaphysical entity like the Soul, or a principle like the pure Ego.

A similar conception, but also a problem, is captured by Dilthey (1976), who draws attention to the difficulty, indeed the impossibility, of completely capturing the flow of life itself. For Dilthey, in sympathy with the views of Heraclitus, the flow of life is 'seeming, but not being, the same, as seeming both many and one' (1976: 210). We cannot capture the sense of flow because, however much we strive to do so and strengthen our awareness of it, 'we are subject to the law of life itself according to which every observed moment of life is a remembered moment and not a flow; *it is fixed by attention which arrests what is essentially flow*' (1976: 210). Indeed, 'there never *is* a present' (1976: 210) because all that we experience as present always contains memory of what has (even just) passed. Thus, this troublesome notion of *self* which James sees usefully conceptualised as the momentary congealing or 'arrest' of the flow of experience is itself still at one remove from the reality of life.

If we turn from these observations to a second focus of concerns in this domain, a positive characterisation of the concrete psycho-social individual is found in that process which such writers as Jung, Barbu and Fromm call *individuation*. For Jung (1945/1953), individuation meant 'becoming a single, homogeneous being'; individuality embraced our 'innermost, and incomparable uniqueness, and implied becoming one's own self'. Individuation was thus a 'coming to selfhood or self-realisation'; the aim of individuation being to 'divest the self of the false wrappings of the persona on the one hand and the suggestive power of primordial images on the other' (1945/1953: 171–2).

With Barbu (1956) and Fromm (1942), the analysis is more directly psychosocial. Barbu treats individuation as the process whereby democracy 'crystallises', mentally, in as many forms as there are individuals in a particular group; a process that makes possible an adjustment to social expectations without loss of self; a loss of self as might be seen, for example, in totalitarian forms of life. Individuation, as the sense of separateness and difference, yet a being-with-others, is seen by Barbu as correlated with particular forms of social organisation: commercial rather than agricultural, societal rather than communal:

> . . . individuation depends upon factors existing in the individual himself. In a democratic society the individual's mental structure is flexible. This makes it possible for him to adjust himself to the social order of his group and to the pattern of communal life and to remain himself at the same time.
>
> (1956: 48)

The foregoing observations represent a coherent, traditional account of the notion of the individual or the self as having something more than just quantitative existence; 'one among many'. Common experience adds to this view, and at the risk of deepening what is for some an illusory perspective on the self, this experience is worth noting.

Our common experience – though sometimes the experience is more profound than calling it common would suggest – provides examples that are not easily discounted in respect of our felt sense of self. Even when our most personal inner experiences are understood in complex social terms by a theorist (for example, Shotter, 1997), we are left with a deep personal sense that something is 'just not right' or is 'left out' when this is done.

The experiences under focus here give rise to a common folk psychology, illustrative rather than explanatory, provocative rather than an argument against this or that in human experiencing. The idea of folk psychology generates considerable controversy, ranging from a denial of its significance and its worth in illuminating our understanding, across an acceptance of a useful overlap between it and scientific psychology, to the understanding of it, too, in terms of a social constructionist perspective (Gergen, 1985, 1989a). We need not engage the specific debate in folk psychology here, a debate captured well in its different positions in O'Donohue and Kitchener (1996). However, it is useful to record some of the common experiences that go to sustain the qualitative sense of self we also appear to experience.

Perhaps most dramatic as an individual experience, in a sense an *individualising* experience (Heidegger, 1927/1978), is that of *death*. This inevitability of life brings to consciousness the reality of our own transience and vulnerability and forces us to face the concreteness of self. Heidegger (1927/1978) has made a great deal of this. Consciousness of one's non-being is, for Heidegger, *the* significant factor in creating individuality and the manner in which one gains a total perspective on one's life, a sense of wholeness. Death indicates one's separateness, one's aloneness; no one can do a person's dying for him or her. The consciousness of personal death extracts one from the inauthentic group and everyday, trivial cares and concerns. While we struggle with questions about this or that possession, friendship, task, personal problem or mood state, we are unable to struggle with, to return to, the question of what it is to *Be*. This awareness of death, moreover, provides the originating impetus for reflection on the world in the first place (Bubner, 1981). Indeed, as far as the social construction of death goes, Heidegger identifies 'the They', other people, as the most significant factor in distracting our attention from the reality of our own deaths and thereby from our individuality. While Sartre (1943/1966) takes issue with Heidegger's specific argument, he nonetheless does not shy away from the significance of death in developing his notion of self, a notion of 'authentic selfhood' based on choosing.

Bereavement also confronts us with a reminder of our individuality and the sense of an isolated self, and it, too, is also significant to Heidegger's analysis (Leman-Stefanovic, 1987). The status of being a bereaved person is associated with the complex reaction that is *grief*. Grief can be variously conceptualised but a useful formulation is that of Switzer (1970). This is in terms of a three-sided anxiety reaction. First, there is anxiety over the loss of a part of oneself that was invested in or identified with the loved, lost object. There is also a moral anxiety, or guilt, over real of imagined failings in relation to the deceased. Third, and importantly here, there is a sense of one's own mortality, a sense of existential or ontological anxiety. While the first two components are more assimilable to group understandings and expectations, the third is less so.

There are also states on the way to death, such as serious illness. When we are ill we are forced to look at ourselves as frail, dependent creatures in which the self struggles against the impersonal, public, institutionalising health-care system. When we are ill our sense of self-esteem is shattered, our self-concept is altered to one that includes dependence, as our cherished independence is lost. Illness forces the perception and acceptance of a new way of being. Moreover, illness itself can be caused by a failure to deal with the self in an honest way, as in Kierkegaard's (1849/1980) 'The Sickness Unto Death', where he discusses the *dread* associated with the realisations about one's self.

There is, finally, the sense we have of ourselves as a continuity, as a story. Crites defends the narrative form as best capturing the 'tensions, the surprises, the disappointments and reversals and achievements of actual temporal experience' (1971: 306), drawing on Augustine's reflections in his *Confessions*. Here, memory is distinguished from recollection. Memory is simply 'storage' of images, whereas recollection is the ordering of memories and the telling of a story based on that ordering.

Now, this notion of our life as a story is where personal construct psychology and the demands of postmodernist thinking in respect of the self most significantly meet with a broader constructivist perspective on the self. We will take this matter up below. First, it is useful to reiterate the current situation in social thought on the self and acknowledge a shift in respect of it.

Decentred and recentred subjects

It is now 'common wisdom' and something of an expanding research paradigm that the notion of a unitary self, of an autonomous, reflective consciousness which relates to the world in an objective way, is no longer tenable. Talk of the self, subjects, 'I', and so forth, is at best illusory, at worst dangerous for clear thinking about, and supportive of, systems of power and oppression. Thus the notion of the decentring of the subject in contemporary philosophy.

This wisdom does acknowledge that there are individuals, but in general, these individuals obey wider laws and are relatively impotent in a context, significantly a social context, which constructs them through language. When some degree of originative behaving is allowed the individual, that is relatively insignificant in the face of external 'laws' impinging on that individual. Thus, while many of the previous observations made about common experiences, and about processes of individuation, would be accepted, they would be deemphasised in favour of impersonal, macro-level forces. This is one reason that such social constructionists as Gergen (1992) reject personal construct psychology at the same time as they champion the idea of 'construction' more generally. Individuals are constructed in and by language, and individuals cannot construct anything significant *personally*.

Interestingly, the most passionate critic of the self or the subject, Michel Foucault, surprised his supporters with a paper late in his career that caused consternation within Foucault scholarship (Foucault, 1982). In this later work he was keen to be seen as developing the relations between three *equal* dimensions of human existence: power, truth and the subject. His earlier work had concentrated too much on one of these, power, and the shift admits the imbalance. As O'Farrell suggests in her account of the shift, 'Foucault explains that the problem with his earlier books was that he had largely ignored the question of "individual conduct"' (1989: 117). Thus, in this paper, 'The Subject and Power', Foucault surprises his disciples and critics alike with observations such as:

> Power is exercised only over free subjects, and only in so far as they are free. By this we mean individual or collective subjects who are faced with a field of possibilities in which several ways of behaving, several reactions and diverse comportments, may be realised. . . . At the very heart of the

power relationship, and constantly provoking it, are the recalcitrance of
the will and the intransigence of freedom.

(1982: 790)

So, there is an obvious individual, but that individual has in the repertoire
of behaviour *several* ways of behaving, *several* reactions, and *several* orientations, positions or significances in respect to even the most pervasive force
acting on the individual, that of *power*. This sounds remarkably like the
process of construing, and, moreover, recalcitrance and intransigence appear
to be remarkable markers of an individual's power to construe in terms of the
fundamental postulate of personal construct psychology and some of its
corollaries.

Constructing selves

As noted above, there have been various attempts to reconstrue the notion of
the self, many of these stimulated by the narrative quality of lived-experience.
Mair (1970b) early on explored this notion via a discussion of an approach to
psychology that favoured a *conversational* approach he was later to develop in
terms of the stories that people form of and in their lives (Mair, 1989). His is a
wider canvas in which he challenges his psychological colleagues to share a
different outlook on the behaving of individuals than they customarily
engage. His challenge is based on his belief that 'we persistently boil down our
experiencing to dull "normality", while our unspoken selves long for a voice
of more passionate precision' (1989: ix). Again, Pocock (1995) has illustrated
a notion of self within this narratological strain, usefully reminding us that
narrative and personal construct approaches, at least, have an idea of some
stories being better than others. This challenges again the charge of relativism
and arbitrariness in personal construct psychology, and strengthens the idea
of differentiating 'real dialogue' from 'idle talk' (Warren, 1992b). Better
stories are suggested to be more congruent, object-adequate, encompassing,
conscious, hopeful, and so forth.

Others have pursued this same narratalogical conceptualisation of the self
within the constructivist approach. Barclay and Smith (1993) examine autobiographical remembering and the manner in which this relates to and
contributes to our sense of self. A metaphor of an 'improvised composition',
as in music, dance or drama, and the like, captures the manner in which the
self is 'composed' in a series of productive acts of remembering, such that 'to
know one's self is to experience directly the compositional process' (Barclay
and Smith, 1993: 20). Compositional activities are seen as bounded by, for
example, cultural, social, historical and psychological factors, providing
thereby resources for the improvisations that go to create a sense of temporal
being.

Balbi (1996) offers a similar account, though using the term *person*. The
essential notion capturing the idea of the person is that of the person as self-

organiser of experience who is aware of its own self-organising, its own subjectivity. To a point, like Chiari and Nuzzo (1996a, 1996b), he follows Maturano and Varela (1987) who centre biological factors, and he finds Gergen's (1991) notion of 'saturation' pertinent but suffering a blind spot. His move beyond the first position and his unease with the second is the result of their failure to give proper regard to the factor of *subjectivity*. Against the first, it is the emergence in primates of an ability to distinguish their own internal states from those of others (shown in the ability to *pretend*, for example) that is the important factor. Against the second, it is the capacity of at least some individuals to *be aware* of the 'saturation' even as it occurs; social constructionists themselves, for example. Thus, he conceives the principal task of psychology as that of understanding 'organized subjectivity' (Balbi, 1996: 260), a particularly apt conceptualisation of psychology for personal construct psychology.

Still within this same vein of the narrative understanding of our lives, Howard, Myers and Curtin (1991) report research studies indicating that individuals can be shown to display self-determination. A crucial factor in this is when the *meaning* of a particular action can be gauged within the more embracing story of their life: 'The stories people live by give meaning to various actions in their lives, and it is the meaningfulness of an action to a person that determines ... the agent's ability to self-determine' (Howard, Myers and Curtin, 1991: 386).

Gonçalves (1995) has developed a similar theme, arguing a notion of self as *project*. He construes life itself as a narrative in which human beings exist through understanding that narrative. Against the metaphor of persons as scientists, he poses the metaphor of persons as dramatic artists, simultaneously interpreting roles of director and actor in life. His approach emphasises one of the three ways in which human beings might be seen to make sense of the world; that is, reason, metaphor and myth (Rowe, 1978). While there may be a difference between claiming life itself as a narrative and our way of dealing with it in terms of stories – Crites' point, with which we began, concerned the narrative quality of our *experience* of the world – Gonçalves' discussion does go to further instance the new conceptions of self emerging from a revitalised constructivist paradigm.

Now, the different accounts of how the self might be understood in alternative terms to that given in the so-called modernist mode of thinking about it can be drawn together to highlight their differences. This task is facilitated here by Cox and Lyddon's (1997) summary. They most conveniently organise the different conceptions of self around five main theories: self-theory, process conceptions, transcendent conceptions, narrative theory and social/economic/political construction.

These different conceptions are unpacked as follows. Self as theory is said to grow from Berzonsky's (1990) reconstrual of Erikson and Marcia's notion of inner identity. A self-theory is a dynamic frame in which experiences are construed. The second idea, self as evolving process, conceives of the self in terms of ongoing action on the world, but action which improves or grows, some say 'evolves', in effectiveness, subtlety or integration – synonyms for the term *process* are *operation, workings, mechanism, procedure,* and the like. This view of self conceives of the self erecting its own identity from interactions in and with the world, especially the world composed of other selves. Bugental (1980) draws attention to the existential dimensions of this view, and Bugental and Bugental (1984) stress the importance of meaning creation as a key element in identity formation.

The third, the transcendent self, alerts us to non-western views, and to the 'self beyond self' of transpersonal psychology. Self as narrative, the fourth view, also emphasises process, but now on a dimension of time. Howard (1991) uses a metaphor of culture as a dynamic backdrop to the story of self, stressing again the impacts, here subtle impacts of context. Elsewhere, Howard had discussed the construct of personal agency, locating the power this implied in a self conceived as a 'center of narrative gravity', analogous to the center of gravity of an object (1986: 168).

Finally there is a view of identity as a composite of different formative ingredients, chiefly social, political and economic. Cushman (1990) and Gergen (1991, 1994) are good examples. For Cushman (1990) self is different in different historical periods, hence must be constructed only by factors identifiable in particular periods. Gergen's 'saturated self' conveys the idea of a sponge which has absorbed a myriad of external influences and which at any point in time is but a collage of these influences. The medium of construction is language, and this, like the test of meaning and the veridicality of an emotion, lies in the community one inhabits.

In terms of this last view, a most sophisticated attempt to account for even our intense inner feelings in social constructionist terms is given by Shotter (1997), not yet included in Cox and Lyddon's summary. His account is a 'rhetorical-responsive version of social constructionism' which suggests that our inner lives are 'neither so private, nor so inner, nor so logical, orderly, or systematic as has been assumed' (Shotter, 1997: 13). While such complex and sophisticated accounts as Shotter's might omit the sense, the lived-experience sense, of something from the innner state associated with real experienced events such as death, illness or bereavement, especially when one is intensely and presently having such an experience, they do indicate the alleged reach of the social constructionist perspective.

Cox and Lyddon (1997) summarise their discussion by indicating the divergences across these five positions and the key matter on which they diverge. That is, while all think in process terms, they differ chiefly in terms of the role of individual *agency*. Those that stress social-political construction are most radical on this score, reducing agency sometimes to a point of disappearance. Neimeyer (1995b) had cast this same set of perspectives on this same dimension, noting a spread from greater agency, through social constructionism, to the annihilation of the self.

The common wisdom, then, is of a generally depreciated notion of self that can be relegated to the sidelines, can be 'decentred'. Yet, what is one to do when a sense of unease results, a sense of 'homelessness' in a previously familiar intellectual climate (Warren, 1997) or of 'misgivings' (Neimeyer, 1995a) in the face of self conceived as 'collage of a randomly assembled relationships' (Neimeyer, 1995a: 351)? Several approaches suggest themselves by way of response in the face of this current common wisdom concerning the self.

One response to the argument that the subject has been discredited is to catalogue the historical attempts to give a substantive account of the self; this simply, but not without significance, restates the thinking underlying the modernist project. A second is to appeal to the common experiences that appear to be devalued in such a decentring, experiences that are to the individual part of a much more important 'lived-experience' of the world; this is 'emotional', but perhaps thereby more rather than less significant to the issue. Still, Shotter (1997) might say that such inner experience *can* be understood in social constructionist terms. A third response is to develop a theory of the self that tries to accommodate the reasonable claims of the social constructionist position. A fourth is to point to shortcomings in the underlying argument for the decentring of the self; that is, idealist social theory that may open up more sinister outcomes in a social relativism.

The first two approaches to the problem are sampled above in references to the efforts of philosophers of the liberal tradition to account for the self, and in some of the common experiences had by the self. The third is more ambitious, and the fourth generates an ongoing debate that could not here be closed.

Nonetheless, at least something needs to be said about the third and fourth responses. As to the third, there are various accounts of the self which chart a course between autonomy and heteronomy and attempt to meet the social constructionist challenge. We have previously noted Colapietro's (1990) statement of the more general pragmatist response to the problem by reworking the notion of personal agency and personal autonomy in a fashion which takes such a course. Colapietro argues, in short, that what is in the currently dominant wisdom's account of the subject is already better contained in pragmatism. In pragmatism, the self is understood as a source of innovation, resistance and creativity. The concept of self as *agent* is stressed by the pragmatists; an agent immersed in formative social contexts, but nonetheless a unique 'centre of action'. For pragmatism, discourse is but another form of communal practice just like any other social experience the individual has. Pragmatism's account stresses what might be expressed as a 'location' or 'grounding' of the self in the lived-ness of everyday life; a view of the self that accommodates the significance of the social without total loss of the self. Further, pragmatism provides a fuller psychology that addresses questions concerning our attending, our thinking, our curiosity. More generally, this response illuminates a 'relational' (Habermas, 1981/1987; Barglow, 1994), a 'dialogical' (Harré and Gillett, 1994; Shotter, 1997), and a 'projectional' (Gonçalves, 1995) notion of self.

Equally, Cox and Lyddon (1997) themselves conclude their summary in terms of the exciting challenges that postmodern thinking throws up for a notion of the self. The emphasis is on self as a dynamic process, on social-cultural context, on interconnectedness, on self as evolving. The constructivist perspectives are concluded to 'offer a paradoxical view of self as constancy through flux, of self defined by other, of self with a center yet intrinsically part of everything else' (Cox and Lyddon, 1997: 217). The echoes of William James here are strong, but also those of personal construct psychology.

The fourth of the suggested responses is to critique the social construc-tionist account of the self. While this is an impossible matter to reach closure on, the types of concerns noted in the previous chapter are relevant to it. That is, that account is, in essence, overextended (Mascolo and Dalto, 1995; Mascolo, Pollack and Fischer, 1997) and perpetuates a relatively passive account of human cognitive functioning (Colapietro, 1990; Rychlak, 1990). Further, it has been argued that it leaves open important technical questions concerning the ontological status of language and the psychological complexity of speech acts (Passmore, 1985). Moreover, the social construc-tionist account deemphasises the importance of individual interpretation and 'making one's own' those cultural 'colorations' that Friedman (1995) refers to as 'touchstones'. Like constructs, which are genuinely one's own, touchstones are insights that 'a person must be willing to test . . . again and again in the "lived concrete"' (Friedman, 1997: 286). Such insights are not to be given up too easily. Further, the general dominant wisdom concerning the decentring of the subject still has to take account of the shift in thinking of one of its significant mentors, Michel Foucault.

Finally, however, we might note a most comprehensive position that merges the last two forms of response, that is, the development of a positive view of the self and a criticism of postmodern views, in a most conciliatory fashion. Frank (1984/1989) identifies *neostructuralism* as a way of mediating between the claims of French poststructuralism and German hermeneutics. In respect of the self, Frank makes *self-acquaintance* a fundamental ontolog-ical given evidenced in our lived-experience, and he attempts to counter the argument that because concepts like 'the subject' and 'subjectivity' are equiv-ocal, they should be liquidated from philosophy. Rather, even while the concept of *self-understanding* as emphasised by hermeneutics has some prob-lems, it is still hardly imaginable that 'we can expect a solution of the problem from an alternative theoretical concept that is founded on the principle of the *non*understanding of itself' (Frank, 1984/1989: 344). Frank's position is captured succinctly and aptly for the present focus of our discussion as follows:

[What was needed was] a theory of the individual subject that internalizes structures in a nonidentical way and reexternalizes them in an altered form . . . This would mean bringing into play a *hermeneutics of individuality* of a sort in which the individual moment is not an opponent, but rather a moment of the structure; that is, a moment of such a type that it prevents the structure from closing itself and thus prevents it from exercising a one-sided determination.

(1984/1989: 358)

A positive notion of self might, then, not only emerge from the debate between modernity, poststructuralism and hermeneutics, but such a notion might be a *necessity* in that debate. Frank's (1984/1989) account goes a considerable way in opening up this and wider matters.

There is a final different point worth making in the present context and derived from our earlier reference to Merleau-Ponty (1945/1962). This is the importance of the human body in Merleau-Ponty's work and how this can be developed into a way of reinstating a concept of self that does not offend the objections brought by postmodern thinking. Taking this further, however, O'Loughlin (1997) finds in Merleau-Ponty's work a way of escaping a view of the self or the subject that is properly discrediting of the autonomous self of modernity, but does not 'degender' the self. She argues that his work provides an account of body-subjectivity that enables a conceptualisation that maintains the female difference that is too easily lost in postmodern thinking about the subject.

The trials and tribulations of the notion of the self will undoubtedly continue and we have but highlighted an ongoing debate in the foregoing observations. It appears equally as absurd to refuse to recognise some originating role for an individual as it is to overlook the impact of social forces. For present purposes, the best that can be expected is that a view of self might emerge from personal construct psychology that is attentive to the most recent discreditings of the self of the liberal tradition. Such a best outcome does appear realisable, particularly when the relatively underemphasised social dimension of personal construct psychology is recalled (Kalekin-Fishman and Walker, 1996). Further, in Foucault's (1993) call for a 'critical ontology' which both recognises and endeavours to go beyond our socio-historical situatedness, there appears to be an invitation for a psychology such as personal construct psychology to contribute to such an ontology. In any event, if matters take us towards the rapprochement that Frank (1984/1989) invites, personal construct psychology may well live up to its characterisation as 'the only psychology for the future' (Rowe, 1996).

All of this said, we can conclude with a consideration of efforts addressed to the notion of the self specifically in personal construct psychology, remembering the references already made in passing above in connection with the narrative quality of experience.

The self in personal construct psychology

Bannister (1983) has specifically examined self from the perspective of personal construct psychology. It is helpful to review what he refers to as but a sketch, commencing with his conclusion. This is that for personal construct psychology self has a holistic quality, and a lot can be said about it 'without at any point making self a special case or creating a mini-psychology around it' (Bannister, 1983: 386). His approach is to consider the notion of self in terms of the fundamental postulate and eleven corollaries.

From the perspective of the fundamental postulate, self is regarded as central in that stream of events which are anticipated by the person. To misconstrue another is a not insignificant concern, but to misconstrue one's self is far more concerning. Thus the confusion and shock when we misread or poorly estimate our own ability and end up in a situation in which we can only conclude we were 'not ourselves' in that particular action or event. In regard to our anticipation of our own behaviour we develop core role constructs which sustain the self. These emerge in our values, our philosophies of life, our hopes for our future, our 'story'. Thus, personal construct psychology identifies *guilt* as an outcome of a failure to predict and understand our actions and the consequent dislodgement of self from the core processes which maintain our personal integrity.

As to the corollaries, the *construction corollary* would suggest that when we interpret common themes in our experience we are not doing this in some disinterested, mechanical fashion, but so as to interpret our lives, Life in general, and our place, the place of our self, in the scheme of things. The *individuality corollary* suggests that there will be a wide array of different selves, selves which know and reflect on their difference from others. The *organisation corollary* indicates that self will be differently located in the construct system for different individuals; that is, for some it will be superordinate, for others peripheral. For example, self may be subordinate to constructions of God or country; in this, cross-cultural differences in regard for the self *vis-à-vis* ancestors or the community generally might be understood. The *dichotomy corollary* indicates that in the construction of self different contrasts will be in operation in different contexts and that understanding self will depend significantly on what in each particular context self is being contrasted with – for example, with not-self when we reflect on the magnitude and mystery of the cosmos; with others when we reflect on interpersonal relationships; with how we see ourselves and how we would like to see ourselves; with the 'me' rather than the 'I' in public situations or in different roles we play. Bannister believes that one failure of orthodox so-called self-psychology is its ignorance of the need to consider to what self is contrasted in different contexts. (Another failure is the attempt of the different self-psychologies to join their ideas and experimental data to a 'broad argument as to the psychological nature of humankind': Bannister, 1983: 379). The *choice corollary* suggests that we will choose the alternative that best elaborates *our* system. There is a 'compass-like dedication' to doing that which we see as appropriate to our nature: 'We strive to behave in ways that represent us because any other behaviour would gravely confuse, not only others, but our *selves*' (Bannister, 1983: 382).

The *range corollary* suggests that self will be used for some to cover a broad range of different selves – a range across James' (1907a) 'I' and different senses of 'me' – while for others it will have a narrower convenience to, say, personal relationships or, we might add, transpersonal experiences. The *experience corollary* indicates variation which Bannister suggests is best illustrated in terms of the mode of construing: preemptive, constellatory, propositional. Thus a self construed preemptively will close off other avenues of construction. Self construed as a 'naughty boy' will exclude construction as a lovable person, a good student or sportsperson. Self construed in constellatory terms will see such a construction as 'naughty boy' necessarily implying such things as worthless, unlovable, a general nuisance. Self construed propositionally will imply nothing more; 'naughty boy' may be understood as 'good boy who on this occasion did a naughty thing'. The *modulation corollary* shows how self will be differently construed in different situations and how easy or difficult this might be. Thus self construed as 'private' might be easily or only with great difficulty construed as 'public'; as 'civilian' easily or with difficulty construed as 'soldier' on conscription to the army. Equally, shifts from student to teacher, from working to being retired, or single to married will be achieved differently by those who have permeable rather than impermeable constructions of self.

The *fragmentation corollary* suggests how my self in different situations may appear totally inconsistent, yet within my system of construing it is quite consistent. The example of the hero of Rhinehart's (1971) provocative novel *The Dice Man* is an example that might have been used to illustrate Bannister's discussion of this corollary in respect to self. Specific behaviours that were indeed random because based on throwing a dice to decide courses of action were in fact based on the hero's ingenious construction of life in terms of the arbitrariness of most if not all of that happens to us. Knowledge of such an overarching construction governing the person's life discloses a consistency in the inconsistency. The *commonality corollary* stresses the importance of others and possible limitations on the elaboration of the self. Thus, we need to elaborate in terms of our contrast with others, and those social systems which encourage conformity will limit the elaboration of self; just as more open societies will expand it. Later, in respect to a consideration of political issues in personal construct psychology, particularly in respect to the psychology of democracy (Barbu, 1956), this will be seen as an indication of an underlying optimism in personal construct psychology. The *sociality corollary* – a corollary that is too easily overlooked and one that is most important to contemporary discussions of the impact of social life on individual construing – stresses, in relation to the self, that we develop our image of ourself by construing other people's constructions of us. Thus is recognised the impact of social meanings on our meanings of self.

Bannister's argument is drawn directly and closely from Kelly, and a view of self from Kelly is illustrative of the general understanding:

> The self is, when considered in the appropriate context, a proper concept or construct. It refers to a group of events which are alike in a certain way and, in that same way, necessarily different from other events. The way in which the events are alike is the self. That also makes the self an individual. The self, having been thus conceptualised, can now be used as a thing, a datum or an item in the context of a superordinate construct. The self can become one of the three or more things – or persons – at least two of which are alike and are different from at least one of the others.
>
> (1955/1991: I, 131/I, 91)

Elsewhere, Bannister drives home the point that the self in personal construct psychology is not socially isolated:

> The distinction between individual man and social man is well lost in construct theory. The theory proposes that our picture of our own individuality is built up by our assessment of others' pictures of us. . . . This makes the individual never less than self-identified by never more than he can understand of others.
>
> (1970: 244)

These quite clear and specific observations noted, we can recall the sympathetic relationship between personal construct psychology and the narrative perspective on self as story (Mair, 1989; Mancuso, 1996a, 1996b). Further we can note other commentary from the perspective of personal construct psychology. Sigel and Holmgren (1983), for example, provide a model of the person that draws on personal construct psychology, merging this with other positions, chiefly those of Piaget and Polanyi. They outline a 'constructive dialectical view' of the person within personality theory. Such a view emphasises 'that we come to know about ourselves through a knowing process', knowing and affect indissolubly linked (Sigel and Holmgren, 1983: 69).

Berzonsky (1989) develops the active notion of the self in terms of a developmental approach to self-identity, stressing again the 'process' nature of the self and providing empirical support for relations between particular construct systems and types of 'self-theorists'. That is, an individual's self-theory is conceived as a set of constructs, schemas, behavioural scripts or strategies that are used to deal with the world. Thus, his notion of 'self as a theorist' as a way of elaborating personal construct psychology: the self active and interactive with the world and formed in this interaction.

A similar account is given by Walker (1990) where the significance of other selves, other persons, is underscored. Other people are the primary sources of elaboration and validation of our construing, and they are particularly important features of the world to 'get right'. In turn, the extent to which selves rely on or depend on one another and the complexities and subtleties of 'dependence' drive home the significance of persons-in-relation in respect to construing the self. Duck (1983) had also emphasised these matters in suggesting the need to build on Kelly's (1955/1991) original formulation of the sociality corollary. In particular, he saw value in reconstruing sociality as 'a complex combination of many levels of thought and behaviour' (Duck, 1983: 41) such that those aspects of another person's construct system which must necessarily be construed might be discerned from those that are less important in social interaction. Mascolo (1994) also calls for an exploitation of the manner in which personal construct psychology is consistent with social constructionism. He expresses the hope that Kelly's ideas might be transformed so as to 'explain how persons and cultures jointly comprise each other' (1994: 103), though he acknowledges that for some personal construct psychologists Kelly can be seen as already accommodating the social dimension. This echoes the development of a notion of a discursive self (Harré and Gillett, 1994) which finds personal construct psychology most congenial, providing that the implicit interpersonal dimension of that psychology is not underconceptualised. This is avoided, in their approach, by insisting on the now familiar point of the location of subjects in discourses. Butt (1996) has also emphasised this dimension of personal construct psychology, arguing that it is this feature of it that removes it from consideration as a cognitive theory. Rather, it is better thought of thereby as a theory of *social action*.

A most insightful perspective on the self for personal construct psychology is provided in Chiari and Nuzzo's (1996a, 1996b) clarification of the different constructivist positions noted earlier. They find particularly strong links between the work of Maturana and Varella (1972/1980) and personal construct psychology in the ideas of an autonomous self-organising system, and structural determinism within the system. This is captured for them best by the notion of *autopoesis*. Generally

> because the functioning of a self-organising system is the expression of its structure of connections, its operations are determined by its structure, not by external inputs having the value of *instructions*. In other words, environment cannot specify the system's changes, but only trigger them, acting as a source of *perturbations*.
>
> (Chiari and Nuzzo, 1996a: 33)

Chiari and Nuzzo (1996a) go on to find in narratologic approaches a way of refocusing personal construct psychology on the more molar level of understanding of the person. This is consistent with their discussion of the manner in which we might see persons as systems enmeshed in other systems, and a mutual interdependence of wholes and parts. Thus, to the question, 'Is mind nothing but brain, or is it a social dimension realised in, but not reducible to, brain, that is, a "higher" (social, cultural, ecological) dimension?', they can answer that it is both.

Now, one particularly interesting aspect of all of this more specific discussion is the manner in which personal construct psychology would appear to already, or relatively easily, accommodate much of the new, and often quite complicated constructions of the self. It would seem to have from the beginning been less sensitive to the attack mounted on the notion of the self by such writers as Foucault (1978/1988, 1982) and the general social constructionist line of thought. As suggested elsewhere (Warren, 1985), personal construct psychology is relatively silent, and relatively neutral, on the origins of individual construct systems. That the individual is 'situated' is perfectly compatible with personal construct psychology, as is the idea of a significant dimension of the 'construction of construction' being the social contexts which the individual inhabits. Again, self as project (Gonçalves, 1995), which is engagingly ambiguous, can be taken as 'projecting', that is, *construing, giving meaning to*, expressing an 'inner outlook'.

What personal construct psychology does want to do, however, is to accord a greater rather than a lesser importance to the individual's role in constructing the world and the self. This is where the different perspectives come into their significant conflict. However, 'conflict' is curious in the present context, and it is perplexing to contemplate just what is in conflict if some of the combatants are, on their own analysis, merely 'collages', 'metaphors', congealings of discourses, and the like.

As with the debate of which the present wider debate appears to be something of a *déjà vu*, what is argued about is the *weight* or *stress* given to the individual. One conclusion drawn from the Marx–Stirner debate, applicable equally to that between Marxism and existentialism, was previously noted. That is, that each represents a different searchlight illuminating a field from a different angle or perspective. This is perhaps again a useful understanding in respect of the self, and depending on what was one's purpose one or other searchlight would become more illuminating.

Concluding comment

There is, clearly, a great deal of development going on in respect of this notion of the self. Various accounts of the self are in evidence, these more or less taking account of deep, qualitative lived-experience that draws the attention of the existential tradition. Arguments that there just is no substantive self are difficult to sustain, making a form of 'self-contradiction'; certainly such positions are not without their difficulties. The question of some sort of 'locus' for the social forces said to be constructing the self, and the capacity for some to at least partly 'escape' that construction, are significant questions for a denial of the self entirely. The apparent capacity of some to escape the totalising impact of the social forces of capitalism was, indeed, a 'cheap shot' thrown against Marx's analysis, but a shot nonetheless. Equally, the implication of some sort of unitary, unified 'society' existing itself as an 'entity' exerting a cause is questionable; it might just be a little more complex than that. Again, so, too, might that link between language and the individual and the group be more complex and differently examined by linguistics than by philosophers (Harris, 1996).

From the personal construct psychology perspective, self is seen as a process, a stream or flow. It is seen in terms of Heraclitus' analogy of the river, or Bergson and his analogy of the 'song'. We do not in considering a river look for the 'bits' or molecules of water that comprise the river, nor ask what holds it together, nor question one ordering of molecules against another. Just as we cannot step into the same river twice, so 'we are and we are not', we are not the same between two successive instants. The notion of the *body* as constantly breaking down, as going through a continuous process of metabolism (destruction in catabolism, renewal in anabolism), is applied by Heraclitus to the depersonalised Soul as to the world at large. Again, with a song or tune where the melody *is* the relation between the notes and one does not ask which particular notes represent the melody. A similar metaphor could be drawn from narrative theory, likening our lives to a 'story'.

The self in personal construct psychology is not, then, some sort of entity that looks at the world objectively, nor some pure subjective rational process aloof from the world it inhabits. Rather it is an active and interactive process of testing constructs in that world. Significantly, it is the world of other selves that is most important to the process of self formation or self-identity, always person-in-relation (Walker, 1990). This last point seems to be significantly lost in much of the debate which comes to focus on the apparent individualistic emphasis in personal construct psychology. Finally, that self is 'embodied', and personal construct psychology has a place for those preverbal constructs that others (Merleau-Ponty, 1945/1962, for example) have seen as somehow more basic to our life, as ontologically prior and exercising a powerful role, a role that is captured in particular by the artist (Johnson, 1993). We live, that is, as much *aesthetically* as in other ways, and this is equally worthy of recognition as is the narrative quality of our experience.

Whatever significance that self has in the wider scheme of things, for example in initiating change or seeing clearly the real state of affairs in domination and oppression, that self can only be given more or less significance, not done away with as a concept. It is equally difficult, notwithstanding the reality of different discourses, to disallow that self some degree of originating significance, more than a simple mediating role but, rather, something more substantial, and perhaps something 'individualising' of experience. Personal construct psychology appears to be well placed to assist efforts to compromise competing claims and not inherently wedded to the particular self of modernity which it had already moved beyond in its own original formulations. In the end, however, personal construct psychology assists such compromises by standing firmly on a view which gives greater recognition to the personal and subjective, and to the self as at least in some respect an agent. It would appear to support any elaboration of the notion of self that does not do damage to these features.

6   Philosophical psychology

There has been a recent resurgence of interest in the relation between philosophy and psychology, addressed especially to problems common to both and which would 'yield only to philosophically sophisticated psychologists or to psychologically sophisticated philosophers' (Block, 1980: I, v). Equally, O'Donohue and Kitchener (1996) find a healthy new interdisciplinary approach in evidence.

This field of interest is variously described as philosophical psychology, philosophical problems in psychology, or the philosophy of psychology; each perhaps subtly different yet addressing similar issues. Quite early on, Harriman (1946) referred to philosophical psychology as the formulation and analysis of basic concepts of psychology, in particular, mind, self, consciousness and cognition. Block (1980: I, 1) defined this domain as 'the study of conceptual issues in psychology', while Corsini's (1994) Encyclopedia refers rather to 'philosophical problems in psychology', summarising these as the problem of the nature of human beings, and the philosophy of science.

It is possible to identify a number of key issues that emerge in discussions within philosophy of psychology, whether one looks to earlier (for example, Brown, 1974) or more recent (for example, O'Donohue and Kitchener, 1996) discussions. The later volume (O'Donohue and Kitchener, 1996) found interest in: epistemology and philosophy of science, behaviourism, cognitive science and philosophical issues in clinical psychology.

We take here four issues and examine where personal construct psychology sits in relation to them: philosophy of science, cognitive science, determinism and free will, and, given the origins of personal construct psychology, philosophical issues in clinical psychology.

Philosophy of science

The philosophy of science has been a significant field of philosophy by reason of the centring of epistemology since Descartes. Various aspects of the general domain of knowledge were considered in some detail in Chapter 1 and it is not necessary to return to them here. The connection between epistemology and philosophy of science is that science, and a particular conception of science, had become the only way to genuine knowledge. Thus, it became important to mark out the territory of science and this necessarily touches upon the notion of psychology as a science.

In recent years, at least since Kuhn's (1970) work, philosophy of science has been something of a 'growth area' in philosophy. Spurred on by a revitalised sociology of knowledge in the late 1960s, a significant critique of science had emerged; to a point where Passmore (1978) was led to ask whether criticism had gone too far. Passmore saw that science was a complex enterprise in what it had become, but essentially simple in its real nature. The first, what it had become, quite properly attracted criticism for the anti-human consequences of science, its pretensions and unintended consequences. The second, the essential nature of science as 'objective', imaginative, individual inquiry, however, was too easily lost, and dogma and superstition reinstated if we 'threw out the baby with the bathwater'. It is sufficient here to note the general thrust of this critique, and that one importance of it was in attacking science as having emerged as the *only* way to resolve the problem of epistemology. It was curious that as developments in philosophy of science were raising significant problems for the physical sciences, psychology was attempting to establish itself as a science. This was chiefly as a science in the same mode of the physical sciences, and drawing on the work of Campbell (1957), who provided criteria that psychology, so it was thought, could meet.

This conception of science in psychology has come under attack in recent times and a more appropriate conception of science for psychology has been argued to lie in a focus not on 'explanation, prediction, and control', but in 'understanding'. This was to produce *verstehen analysis*, an approach to the science of human beings that grows out of phenomenology and whose purpose was to understand *human* phenomena in a manner different to the way natural phenomena were to be approached. Vico and Dilthey are particularly relevant theorists for this view.

This last shift is more germane to our purposes here and Bannister and Fransella's characterisation usefully sets a tone for the placement of personal construct psychology in this domain of philosophy of science:

> . . . it presents us with a framework which is cousin to history and poetry, while embodying the kind of systematic attack, public definition and experimental articulation which are the universal aspects of science. It is a psychological theory which admits that values are implicit in all psychological theories and takes as its own central concern the liberation of the person.
>
> (1971: 12)

Two particular discussions provide two different accounts of how philosophy of science can be understood for personal construct psychology. One derives from Rychlak (1968/1985), the other from Warren (1990a).

First, Rychlak (1968/1985) has not only provided a comprehensive discussion of the philosophy of science for personality theory, but has done so with particular reference to personal construct psychology. In outlining the dimensions of a theory of personality, any theory of personality, Rychlak adopted a particular 'image of man'; an adoption he suggests is inescapable. That is, while not attempting to write a theory of personality, his discussion cannot escape putting forward at least an outline of how human beings as a species might look from the point of view of a good theory of personality. He identifies eight features of the image of the human being that inform his discussion.

These features summarise as follows. Human beings bring to experience an existing set of categories such as 'self-concepts, phenomenal fields, life lines, personal constructs, the stereotypes of an authoritarian bigot', and so on (Rychlak, 1968/1985: 470). Experiencing of the environment is at base a search for meaning; the framework of stored meaning with which new experience is approached is to be *extended*, not merely tended. Stored information, memory, is not to be likened to a passive stockpile, but is 'worked over' through a process of *reflection*; moreover, this can be a process of *self*-reflection. The beginning of volitional action lies in a tension – a dialectical opposition – which can initiate a response or course of action that neither of the alternatives in tension was offering. Such response or course of action can become an 'ought' which, projected onto a situation, develops what we know as 'values'; when these responses are shared across individuals, we see the operation of group values which serve as significant controllers on behaviour. While that dialectical reasoning in which individuals cannot escape engaging leads to creative, perhaps unique understandings, not all reasoning is so innovative; thus, consistencies in behaviour are observed and can be used to predict future behaviour within the bounds of different levels of statistical probability. Emotions enter this picture in terms of the human being's capacity or inclination to hang on to established understandings in the face of challenge; 'he strives to cling to the meanings he wants to believe rather than accepting others' (1968/1985: 473). Finally, the possibilities that an individual has self-reflectively arrived at can be made real in behaviour; an individual can cling to his or her position 'long enough to occasionally "make it so" in his life' – the person of conviction, the moralist, the revolutionary or the zealot, committed to a final cause which is proven by and through his or her own life (1968/ 1985: 473).

In summary, then, Rychlak has provided an account of a philosophy of science for personality theory, outlining what an adequate science of personality should include or address. In turn, he finds personal construct psychology extremely well placed in including or addressing all of the matters he prized. Elsewhere (Rychlak, 1978) he suggests the 'dialectic' nature of personal construct psychology, a view he amplifies (Rychlak, 1977/1988) when expressing the hope that such a focus will not be lost.

The second, related direction for placing personal construct psychology in terms of a congenial philosophy of science is, as elsewhere suggested (Warren, 1990a), that personal construct psychology is an example of what Kurt Lewin

(1931, 1935) called the Galileian mode of thought in psychology. This mode of thought stressed *processes* rather than categories and Lewin felt that it was because psychology had moved from philosophy via medicine and pedagogy that it had remained with the Aristotelian mode of thought, to its detriment.

The difference between an Aristotelian and a Galileian mode of thought in psychology is as follows. The Aristotelian mode of thought proceeds by *imposing* on phenomena or events to be understood or explained some predetermined concepts that purport to provide the logical categories into which that phenomenon or event falls. These are fixed categories, unaffected by situations or contexts; around one-quarter of Aristotle's surviving works deal with biology, one of the most taxonomic of the sciences. These fixed factors or vectors are derived initially from empirical observation of what is common to, for example, food getting, fighting or mutual aid. These factors are then set up as, for example, instincts, which function then as explanatory entities to account for hunting, aggression or cooperation.

The Galileian mode of thought, by contrast, sets out to ascertain the factors operating in a particular behaviour and to explain that behaviour in terms of the *interaction* of those factors. There is no idea of fixed types or categories. So flexible is this last feature, in fact, that the factors relevant to a particular situation are themselves seen as variable; for example, they interact and each can be changed. Lewin's example is of a child equally attracted at the same time to a toy and to a piece of chocolate. Internal factors not immediately involved in this particular attraction are drawn into the situation and these and the original motives are all changed as the child realises that both toy and the chocolate cannot be obtained. Thus the two 'motives' or 'wishes', here for toy and chocolate, interact and lead to an outcome that would not be predicted if one was not aware of how they interact with other needs and wants in the total life space. That is, that whole situation changes with the interaction of the factors that are introduced by the realisation of the impossibility of satisfying both wants. Also changed is the strength and direction of the vectors that at every moment are determining the dynamics of the particular field of individual-in-situation. This is akin to Rychlak's point above about 'dialectical reasoning': the outcome of a choice between two alternatives might well be something that is a 'synthesis' of both of them in the sense of something altogether different from, yet related in a generative sense to, each of those alternatives. It is akin also to a more satisfactory account of causation, one which recognises the significance of the field in which causes operate.

The focus of concern for the Galileian mode of thought is the individual case, unlike the Aristotelian mode of thought, which treats this as a phenotype. That is, it is regarded in terms of obvious, visible characteristics that link it to its type; a phenotype involves grouping in terms of shared 'origins'. The Galileian mode of thought looks rather to what might be obscured by too ready a focus on obvious characteristics that might in fact highlight merely superficial similarities; such as in the example of authoritarian mentality where quite different behaviours, such as those associated with doctrinaire communism and its trenchant opposition in fundamentalist Catholicism or fascism, share the same underlying dynamic and appear as but species of this underlying personality type or underlying construct system.

Personal construct psychology, then, perpetuates an approach that in terms of method and theory stands at the forefront of forward thinking about how the quest for understanding in the domain of human behaving is best conducted. This last 'best' is in terms of a recognition of the special approach required to the special 'object' of study that is human behaving. It is also in terms of a recognition of the importance of according a special integrity to that object of study. Moreover, as previously noted, it is addressed to human *behaving* (Koch, 1973) rather than *behaviour*; thus recognising the importance of willing, wishing, hoping, dreaming and other features of human life that are lost in a focus on observable 'behaviour'. In this approach, too, personal construct psychology expresses the orientation provided by Dilthey in his insistence on a different method of approach for studies in the human as against the natural sciences, a differentiation already foreshadowed by Vico. Whatever the ultimate adequacy of this differentiation philosophically (Gadamer, 1960/1975), it would appear to be a useful one for psychology to bear in mind. This is especially so if the methods applicable to the natural sciences do not bear fruit in psychology generally, as is arguably the case.

Finally, personal construct theory has an interesting position in philosophy of science because of its *reflexivity* and, importantly its *disposability* or *expendability*. The broad range of convenience of the theory extends to the issue of how human beings operate on the world to produce theories in the first place. This includes personal construct theory itself. Hence its reflexivity, but also its particular placement in illuminating the very activity of theory-making. Further, there is a recognition that personal construct psychology does not represent some sort of absolute or eternal truth about human functioning; that is, it is disposable. In this respect we are reminded of earlier observations concerning Stirner's insistence that no abstract concept be held so firmly that it cannot be given up, no concepts reified such that they own us more than we own them.

Cognitive science

The relationship between personal construct psychology and Cognitive Psychology has been, perhaps surprisingly, a vexing matter. This is complicated further by the use of capitals to distinguish a fully fledged position in psychology developed in the late 1960s and early 1970s (for example, Neisser, 1967, 1976) in direct opposition to the other main contenders, psychoanalysis and behaviourism, from the study of processes of thinking, memory, problem-solving, and the like. Thus Cognitive Psychology, a position, might be differentiated from cognitive psychology, a focus on processes. The matter of the relationship between personal construct psychology and Cognitive

Psychology developed in fact into something of a 'movement' for integration, one in which personal construct psychology was seen as either one type of 'cognitive position', or a position which embraced, as in the sense of 'incorporates' the cognitive perspective.

Whatever the present state of play in respect of it, the surprising aspect of this development for integration is that Kelly (1955/1991) had initially written consistently and insistently against being labelled as a 'cognitive psychologist'. The Kelly references concerning the illegitimacy of the linkage with cognitive psychology are by now well known (see, for example, Adams-Webber, 1990; Fransella, 1995; Warren, 1990b, 1991). Equally, the integrationist perspective is well documented (for example, Holland, 1970; Neimeyer, 1985, 1988). Jahoda (1988) tried to defuse the developing tensions by drawing attention to a shift in meaning of the concept of 'the cognitive', though Rychlak (1978, 1968/1985) would want to see any such shift had avoided the mechanistic, 'efficient-cause' notion of theorising about human psychological functioning; that is, not merely a methodological shift had occurred, but a paradigmatic one.

What is of greater interest under the present heading and in terms of present more general interests, is the development of cognitive science which claims as one of its progenitors, the discipline that is philosophy, as well as findings in cognitive psychology, if not the theoretical position that is Cognitive Psychology. Cognitive science developed in the 1970s and is of mixed pedigree. It is an interdisciplinary field in which cognitive psychology, linguistics, philosophy, anthropology and artificial intelligence research (the concept of artificial intelligence already itself an assumption of the field) combine to focus on human functioning.

Gardner (1985) provides a history of the so-called 'cognitive revolution', identifying five paramount features of a cognitive science perspective. These summarise as follows. That in discussion of human cognitive functioning it is necessary to work with some conceptualisation of *mental representation*, which operates at a level separate from both the biological and the social. That the computer serves as the most viable model of, as well as an indispensable tool for studying, human mental functioning. That in the short term, and mainly for strategic purposes, certain factors have to be ignored as complicating the enterprise. That advances in understanding significantly involve interdisciplinary cooperation. Finally, that the tradition in which cognitive scientists work and the domain they seek to illuminate is the epistemological; a domain whose basic questions as raised initially by the ancient Greeks still enervate this field. The third, strategic, point may have weakened somewhat since the mid-1980s; that is, that that functioning which is under scrutiny now not only includes our problem-solving but, from some approaches within cognitive science at least, our valuing, our ethical outlooks, our development of ideals (Hooker, 1995, 1996).

In one sense the present discussion of personal construct psychology is in a 'no lose' situation in respect of these matters. If, as proponents of a more 'cognitive view' argue, successfully, personal construct psychology is consistent with the most satisfying theoretical position in cognitive science, then that underscores the philosophical dimensions of the theory being articulated here. If it emerges that personal construct psychology is outdated by a more satisfying theoretical position, then personal construct psychology itself accommodates this in terms of Kelly's (1955/1991) own encouragement to use and then move on from it.

These observations allow us to bypass the issue of whether or not personal construct psychology 'is' cognitive. It is better to say that it contains concepts, methodologies and, importantly, an 'image of persons' that are consistent with the most advanced thinking in cognitive science; and provides a 'psychology for' cognitive science in any of its modes (naturalistic or mechanistic, for example). The fine-grain of cognitive science was worked out long after personal construct psychology had appeared. Interestingly, however, Kelly (1955/1991) was himself not dismissive of the value of applying ideas developing in one area in another, and he makes an observation pertinent to the present discussion of cognitive science: 'The notions of cybernetics and servo-mechanisms have represented useful exchanges between physics and psychology' (Kelly 1955/1991: I, 185/I, 129).

A cursory look at the literature of cognitive science finds it relatively blind to the cautions that Neisser (1976) had raised. More generally, cognitive science is obviously not unproblematic and may raise as many issues as it has been able to resolve (Pribram, 1986; Putnam, 1987; Rychlak, 1991b). It may also represent an integration that is a 'wrong synthesis' and a 'wrong reduction' (Bunge and Ardila, 1987: 273). However, while contemporary critics literate in both psychology and philosophy find reason to continue to raise problems for cognitive science, our interest is not to evaluate it. Rather, the task here is to give a coherent account of where cognitive science is 'at', and how personal construct psychology relates to the most promising of its lines of inquiry and understandings of psychological functioning. We can take two very useful sources for the attempt to briefly review the field: collections edited by O'Donohue and Kitchener (1996), and Hameroff, Kaszniak and Scott (1996).

O'Donohue and Kitchener suggest that cognitive science shifted philosophy of psychology to a metaphysical orientation with a significant focus on 'issues surrounding the philosophy of mind (together with correlative issues in the philosophy of language)' (1996: 157). They locate one major reason for this in the fact that the earlier dominance of methodological behaviourism had seen the major issues as *epistemological* (questions about the behavioural evidence for the existence of minds), but that the cognitive revolution forced a return to questions concerning the nature of the mind that is doing the knowing. Cognitive science, for them, is thus primarily an attempt to understand the knowing mind, and the dominant model for understanding emerged as a *computational* model. This model relies on an idea of 'encoding', a notion that information is gathered in perception, encoded in a fashion that makes cognition possible, and cognition occurring in terms of language. The metaphor is that of a computer processing information by coding and recoding. An alternative model, a *connectionist* model, conceives of parallel processing of encoded information. This is a more complex and sophisticated understanding but one which still draws critics.

What is significant here is that notable alternative positions to the computational model involve a conception of mind as 'constituted of natural phenomena in the world, rather than as some supernatural intrusion into the world' (Bickhard, 1996). Similarly, Hooker (1996) offers a further elaboration of a naturalist position that emphasises more than a simple encoding and computation, but which recognises self-organisation and self-modification.

The second source, the Hameroff, Kaszniak and Scott (1996) volume, is a substantial collection of papers selected from those given in 1994 at the first Tucson Conference titled 'Toward a Scientific Basis for Consciousness'. The papers span a wide array of topics and issues and the volume represents a comprehensive sourcebook of advanced thinking in this field. Several of these papers are of interest to the present attempt to gain a succinct overview of the field.

The volume opens with considerations in the philosophy of mind. In this area, the tensions between an account in terms of the activity of brain, on the one hand, and the richness of our subjective experience of consciousness, on the other, remain. As Hameroff, Kaszniak and Scott indicate in their introductory comments, more than a century after William James' reflections, 'although far better informed about the brain and benefiting from the insights of computers [*sic*], we are faced with the same stark choice of dualism and reductionism' (1996: 1). This and other matters are dealt with by subsequent contributors.

Chalmers (1996) distinguishes the *hard* and the *easy* questions in respect of consciousness. The first can be approached with benefit using the range of techniques now available. These include explanation of matters such as differentiating sleep and wakefulness, our capacities for discrimination and categorisation, or our ability to access our own internal states. The hard problems centre on our subjective experience of what is going on when we are experiencing something. Stressed in his guide for an adequate theory of consciousness are a number of principles that are significant in personal construct psychology. Stubenberg (1996) discusses *qualia* – the 'colours, sounds, smells, tastes, tickles, pains in which we are constantly immersed' – for the light they throw on consciousness. He locates his general position as *neutral monism* and discusses *percepts*, 'the immediately known events, examples of which are "patches of colour, noises, smells, hardness, etc. as well as perceived spatial relations"' (1996: 47). These percepts are taken as instances of the phenomenal properties that are *qualia*, and are, in turn, seen as primary, not derivative from properties of the physical world.

Flanagan (1996) discusses dreams, and his complex neurobiological analysis leads to a notion of dreaming as an attempt by the mechanism of the brain to interpret the 'noise' that is sensory input in terms of preexisting structures of meaning: 'Your dreams are expressions of the way you uniquely cast noise that someone else would cast differently' (Flanagan, 1996: 82). Moreover, dreams are related to the more general enterprise of self-knowledge: 'we have learned to use the serendipitous mentation produced by a cortex working with the noise the system produces to further the project of self-knowledge and identity location' (1996: 82). Galin's (1996) insistence on the significance of subjective experience redirects him also to William James. James' account of two types of experience, one definite, the other vague – the nucleus and the fringe – is elaborated for its value to reflection on consciousness and mind. Fringe experience is not conscious and is illustrated in James' examples: 'feelings of familiarity; feelings of knowing; feelings of action tendency (for example, the intention to say so-and-so); expectant feelings (the commands, "wait", "look", "hark"), elicit distinct feelings of the domain from which a new impression is to come' (Galin, 1996: 123). James is found important for drawing attention to what Galin believes, with others in the volume, is missing in accounts of awareness, consciousness, mind: 'the qualitative differences among the elements that constitute subjective experience' (1996: 125). Galin argues that an adequate theory of awareness must include accounts of subjective experience, of 'the feeling of meaning'.

Now, in these observations of some of many contributions, we have indeed been selective. However, so as to allay suspicions that the conclusion that follows is entirely contrived, we can note the view of those who took account of all the papers, and more. The introductory remarks, and the overview and review remarks at various points, repeat several themes. A preliminary comment, however, is to note some remarks of Hameroff, Kaszniak and Scott (1996) by way of their informal impressions and final summation. Informal remarks such as that the problem of consciousness was not solved by the conference, nor were matters 'spinning out of control', but rather there was ground for optimism in 'a time of great intellectual excitement' and interdisciplinary cooperation (Hameroff, Kaszniak and Scott, 1996: xi–xii). Their concluding summation was that there was a remarkably diverse spectrum of views within the scientific community concerning what is known as consciousness, and that, consequently, science does not have a collective opinion on the matter.

As to the themes derived from the varied contributions, two are interesting here. The first was the return of consciousness and mind as respectable topics for scientific research and discussion. The second, perhaps more important here, is the continued recognition of the importance of the *subjective*. That is, the recognition in cognitive science of the need to take account of individual variation, ingenuity and originality in the manner in which information from outside and inside the system is dealt with. This is not 'mere subjectivity', recognised as 'error variance', but an integral and important aspect of cognitive functioning. The comfortable fit of very many of the ideas in this volume with personal construct psychology is noteworthy. What personal construct psychology does, of course, is to come at the phenomena under attention in cognitive science in a different way; that is, a *psychological* way.

One of the more vigorous explorations of the relationship between cognitive science and personal construct psychology occurred from one side of a debate concerning the possibilities for integration between Cognitive Psychology and personal construct psychology (Adams-Webber, 1990; Warren, 1990b, 1991). While the specific interchange may have been at cross-purposes (Fransella, 1995), Adams-Webber (1990) cited a range of work in which basic principles of personal construct psychology had been applied to central problems in cognitive science. Kelly was also said to have presaged some of the fundamental issues in this field and the work of a number of psychologists, philosophers and computer scientists working on those issues said to contribute to an elaboration of personal construct psychology.

This last contention was equally as forcefully taken up in a criticism of Rychlak's (1991a, 1991b) understanding of the relationship between artificial intelligence research and personal construct psychology (Ford, Hayes and Adams-Webber, 1993). The argument was that Rychlak (1991a, 1991b) had misrepresented, or misunderstood, the nature of the 'processing' that was going on in artificial intelligence and that, contrary to Rychlak, such processing was not merely mediational but could be understood as predicational.

It would be foolish here to stray into this last specific debate, but one point is worth making. This is that there are recognised different forms of artificial intelligence. Good old-fashioned artificial intelligence, GOFAI, is criticised within cognitive science in both its narrow (syntactic) version, as well as in its wider (semantic) version. Such criticism has led to better accounts being offered, emphasising biological or evolutionary aspects (Bickhard, 1996; Hooker, 1996). The older version is criticised within the field because of its 'computational' and 'encodingist' assumptions, and the better accounts overcome this by focusing on such things as self-organisation and self-regulation, problem-solving, and the like, all 'wedded to a more connectionist architecture of the mind [moving again] toward the realm of praxis' (O'Donohue and Kitchener, 1996: 158). It is possible that Rychlak (1991a, 1991b) is addressing the older version, while Ford, Hayes and Adams-Webber (1993) are responding in terms of one or other of the newer versions; though they do not cite references that elaborate such versions.

Clearly, these last specific matters are complex, but even given this as well as the absence of a generally accepted viewpoint in cognitive science, we can suggest that personal construct psychology is not at variance with the most advanced thinking in this area. Whether the research and reflection in the domain is an advance on what personal construct psychology offers by way of psychological understanding, the matters that have emerged are entirely comfortable for personal construct psychology. Adams-Webber (1990) and Ford, Hayes and Adams-Webber (1993) are correct in this respect as long as they express the matters in terms of complementarity rather than integration.

Either both are theories of the *Logos* and thus complementary in terms of illuminating the same questions but differently. Or, on the other hand, one is from the *Bios* and the other from the *Logos*, in which case, we have again two searchlights illuminating the same territory.

In this vein, we might recall Kelly's (1955/1996) own caution concerning the matter of demarcating *psychological* from other types of theories. The key ideas in his discussion are those of the 'foci of convenience' and the 'range of convenience'. The range of convenience refers to the 'expanse of the real world over which a given system or theory provides useful coverage'. The focus of convenience is the point at which a given theory is particularly applicable (1955/1991: I, 17–18/I, 13). Kelly clarifies this with reference to three theories: stimulus–response theory had a particular focus on animal learning, field theories on human perception, and psychoanalytic theories on human neurosis. Generally, however:

> There is no clear criterion by which a theory can be labelled 'psychological', and not 'physiological' or 'sociological'. There is much interrelationship. The stimulus–response theories in psychology bear a close family resemblance to the interaction theories of physiology. There are field theories in physiology which resemble the psychology of Gestalt. Whether a theory is called 'psychological', 'physiological', or 'sociological' probably depends upon its original focus of convenience.
>
> (1955/1991: I, 18/I, 13)

In these terms, then, one would have to ask what personal construct psychology might contribute to cognitive science and what might it learn from it? The shift to concerns with 'mind' find a congenial account of the way in which mind *operates*, rather than what it is. This may well assist cognitive science through the same type of input made by Cognitive Psychology and research on cognitive processes. Indeed, the refusal of personal construct psychology to follow the classical and deceptive threefold classification of mind into cognitive, affective and volitional processes would seem to broaden the contribution beyond what Cognitive Psychology might offer.

There is one particularly original development that illustrates these last points most elegantly. It also offers an extension of the focus of personal construct psychology itself. This is the work of Rychlak (1991a, 1994, 1996) and his co-workers (Rychlak *et al.*, 1989; Rychlak, Stilson and Rychlak, 1993). Rychlak (1994) develops what he calls logical learning theory as a way of understanding learning which pays proper regard to the predictional manner in which individuals approach the world, and to *all* of the causal factors differentiated by Aristotle. Rychlak (1996) sketches his argument for a non-mechanical model of human functioning which stresses teleology, and he coins a term *telosponsivity* to capture the idea of 'action-intentions' framed by the individual (Rychlak, 1994: 153). The *telosponse* is defined in terms totally sympathetic to personal construct psychology: 'A *telosponse* is the affirmation or taking of a position regarding a meaningful content (image[s], word[s], judgmental comparison[s], etc.) relating to a referent acting as a purpose for the sake of which behaviour is then intended' (1994: 153).

In a series of experiments emerging from this style of thinking about cognition, the notion of *oppositionality* has been explored empirically (Rychlak *et al.*, 1989). Oppositionality was understood as a process that was naturally occurring in the cognitive processing of human beings, 'a necessary or natural tie of one meaning to its contrary or contradiction, even though this tie may not be readily apparent or expressed overtly by the person concerned' (Rychlak *et al.*, 1989: 181–2). A series of experiments demonstrated the advantage given to learning by adopting a strategy of oppositionality in a learning task. Again, the idea of *predication* in human learning was demonstrated in another series of experiments (Rychlak, Stilson and Rychlak, 1993). Predication is the process whereby meaning is extended from a broader to a narrower context. These experiments also went to support Rychlak's logical learning theory, the claim that 'ongoing cognition involves the continued "taking of a position" within a sea of opposite possibilities' (1994: 479).

The last experiments challenge the promise of such areas as artificial intelligence when this is based on a computer model of mind. Rychlak turns his attention to an analysis of issues in artificial intelligence arguing that there was an 'essential side to our natures that artificial intelligence is missing' and that if we pursue the computer analogy too far we distort our human agency (1991: 161).

Throughout all of the discussions in the field of cognitive science what is highlighted repeatedly – in addition to that discussion legitimising notions of mind and consciousness – is the significance of subjective experience and the subjective meaning of experience. Personal construct psychology offers the most thoroughgoing approach to understanding the human meaning-making process and of elaborating the structures of meaning emerging in the individual, whatever their origin.

Bickhard's (1993) observation is an apt one with which to conclude this section: 'constructivism . . . is simply the way the world is – it is how epistemology must work, and any research program with epistemological aspirations, such as artificial intelligence, that ignores it will do so at severe cost' (1993: 276).

Determinism and free will

This is perhaps a less significant issue in current philosophical psychology but worth comment given that Kelly (1955/1991) devotes attention to it. He distinguishes two kinds of determinism, at least for his purposes: that envisaged by his own theory as applying between subordinate and superordinate constructs, and that which might hold in or of the universe. In respect of the latter, the notion of an integral (that is, a complete or whole) universe is that in which there is a flow or an essential continuity. Thus, because 'of this continuity we may consider that there is determinism operating between antecedent and consequent events' (1955/1991: I, 20/I, 15). This second sense of determinism is considered relatively unimportant to his *psychology*, though it is taken as a given, as in the realist position previously outlined.

In respect to the more important aspect of determinism, Kelly's (1955/1991) thinking appears to be in accord with a pluralistic understanding of determinism that rejects the monistic view of causal chains linking things, events, and so on, and replaces it with a notion of causes operating in *fields*. We considered this previously in Chapter 3. Determinism in the pluralist sense that is important to realism conceives of every event in the world having a cause, the world as composed of things, events or situations which both determine and are determined by others. However, it is not a matter of looking to a cause X for event Y, but of looking to the context or field in which that interaction took place; in a different field a different event might be observed.

In so far as personal construct psychology is concerned, this might be understood as follows. Every event or situation is determined, that is, has causes or determinants. However, there is no fixed, common determinant. Rather, what is efficacious will depend on the field in which different potential determinants are operating. If the construct system is understood as a 'field', then a particular other situation or event will be more or less efficacious as a determinant in that construct system depending on its state *vis-à-vis* the determinants operating. Bannister and Fransella (1971) use an example to explain 'anxiety' in personal construct psychology terms. Anxiety occurs when we do not have appropriate constructs to use in a situation in which we find ourselves. Thus, in their example, sex will cause anxiety for the chaste, 'books for the illiterate, power for the humble, and death for nearly all of us' (1971: 35). Moreover, there is an additional determinant in the field's own natural dynamic of striving to continue its own integrity and/or a continued elaboration. This introduces a dimension of intentionality, that is, a *formal cause* element.

This matter of determinism is taken up by Chiari and Nuzzo (1996a) as a way of understanding personal construct psychology in terms of Varella's (1979) account of self-organising systems. In such systems, both determined and autonomous levels are discerned, analogous to Kelly's (1955/1991) account of determinism and freedom as 'two complementary aspects of structure. They cannot exist without each other' (1955/1991: I, 78/I, 55). Rather, a 'thing is free *with respect to something*; it is determined *with respect to something else*' (1955/1991: I, 78/I, 55). We might compare this statement with one made by Anderson: 'Psychological science will only be possible if we have a variety of psychological truths, between which, and in each of which, connection and distinction are discernible' (1962: 14).

There is also a negative aspect to determinism, noted by Kelly, however. This is found in Kelly's (1962b/1979) discussion where he notes how a broad stimulus-response approach to understanding human behaving adopts a determinism which looks only to antecedent factors in a particular behaviour;

the belief 'that one event is bound to lead to another' (1962/1979e: 202). If genuine understanding is sought, however, we must look to a different type of determinism. This is one which at one level sees superordinate constructs determining others, but also, and more importantly, constructions themselves determining behaving. There is in this view a position close to what Anderson commends of Freud's work: its insistence on the definiteness of mental connections, on 'mental mechanism or determinism in terms of which alone there can be a study of human character or a human character to study' (Anderson, 1962: 361).

It would seem, then, that personal construct psychology had from the outset a coherent position in respect of the issue of determinism. Further, such a position is intelligible in terms of, and prophetic for, advanced contemporary thinking about the operation of self-organising systems.

Philosophical issues in clinical psychology

The particular place of clinical psychology, as practice, in personal construct psychology is taken up in the next chapter, which is addressed to 'psychotechnology'. There, it will be argued that personal construct psychotherapy is rather a *praxis* than a practice, Here, however, it is useful to note two specific issues that have particularly worried philosophers: the concept of 'mental illness', and classification and categorisation of mental disorder.

In regard to the concept of mental illness, the main concern has been the relatively arbitrary manner of its delineation, and, related to this, the manner in which the right to determine mental illness is accorded to the power elites of society (Foucault, 1961/1977).

In personal construct psychology the term 'optimal psychological functioning' is used to convey the ideas that the more difficult notion of 'mental health' sought to convey. By contrast, mental illness would be understood as less than optimal functioning, though some notion of 'degree' of deficiency becomes important. Raskin and Epting (1993) have systematically examined the manner in which personal construct psychology offers a more satisfactory account of matters raised by Szasz (1974) in his concept of the myth of mental illness. Their account shows how personal construct psychology is inconsistent with a 'mental illness' approach to psychological problems, reinforcing the opposite approach that emphasises optimal functioning.

Landfield (1980) proposed a dimension ranging from *chaotic fragmentalism* across *perspectivism* to *literalism* as a way of contrasting modes of relating one's feelings, values and behaviour and a way of understanding mental health as optimal functioning. In general terms, the literalist has an overly 'tight' relation between feelings, values and behaviour, the perspectivist a more moderate degree of linkage, and the fragmentalist an extremely loose connection.

Leitner (1982) developed this dimension and provided a succinct example of the three modes of construing along the following lines. A married person might be sexually attracted to the partner of a good friend. As a literalist 'to think it is to do it' and thus for this person adulterous behaviour has been engaged in, which offends his or her values concerning what a good friend and a good spouse is. Guilt and anxiety are experienced. The perspectivist, on the other hand, can acknowledge the aroused feelings, choose to act on them or not, and if values are in place concerning fidelity in both friendship and marriage, find higher-order constructs that might override these and rationalise the action. Finally, the fragmentalist might act by making an impulsive sexual gesture and, despite holding strong values concerning fidelity, not see the most promiscuous behaviour as a negation of them. Generally, the work on this dimension has focused on the two extremes, though Epting and Amerikaner's (1980) account of 'optimal functioning' addresses the midpoint, perspectivism. Further, Button (1985) discusses the related idea of 'psychological well-being', stressing social context factors.

From the point of view of matters arising from philosophical aspects of clinical psychology, then, these observations highlight an important point. This is that the focus on mental health, on optimal functioning, was from the start a feature of personal construct psychology. This suggests a relative immunity to much of the attack from critics concerned with the relatively arbitrary application of the label 'mental illness' and to a congenial place for personal construct psychology in a contemporary context which has found wellness rather than illness a more appropriate focus of attention.

The second point, the categorisations and classifications of so called mental illness, has attracted criticism in general, and specific criticisms of specific attempts to do so in such systems as the early *DSMs* (*Diagnostic and Statistical Manual of Mental Disorders*) and *ICD-10* (*International Classification of Disease*, 10th revision) (Sadler, Wiggins and Schwartz, 1994); these are additional to any difficulties personal construct psychology might have with such classification (Sarbin and Mancuso, 1980). While the axiological approach of the later *DSMs* goes some way toward meeting some of the criticism, this approach continues to suffer from the tension between 'scientific and practical' that leaves the *DSM* open to a variety of problems in respect of which there is 'no consensus and no definitive answers' (Sadler, Wiggins and Schwartz, 1994: 12).

Interestingly, all of the outstanding problems for the future of the *DSMs* as identified by these last writers have significance for a personal construct psychology approach. Thus, the question 'What are they?' of psychiatric diagnoses addresses their mixed pedigree as scientific, evaluative and practical. This question might be responded to by personal construct psychology – in an attempt to be helpful and despite strong reservations about classification – by seeing such diagnoses as hypotheses, tools or aids and as attempts by professionals to construe the construction processes of another person. The issue of the boundaries between mental disorder and mental health can equally well be responded to in more 'continuous' and benign terms by personal construct psychology as a naturalistic psychology. And the criticism of older philosophy of science and its dualisms is familiar to personal construct psychology. Again, the multifaceted connections between psychiatry – and so-called applied psychology – and society is no surprise to personal construct psychology, which has inbuilt modes of understanding this connection. Moreover, the operation of superordinate constructions on the very exercise of developing these classification systems themselves provides a disclosure of ideological as well as 'scientific' imperatives in those classificatory systems (Sarbin and Mancuso, 1980).

More specific to this second matter of classification, personal construct psychology has had from the beginning a scepticism concerning classification. Kelly (1965/1979j) devoted a specific consideration to classification in psychiatry and psychopathology. Generally, classification was considered an obstacle to theory development, that is, to understanding. Further, it was too easily overlooked how what we 'impose' when we classify so easily comes to be seen as what we 'find' in the phenomena of concern to us. Categorisation, moreover, imposes restraints that later are extremely difficult to overcome; and 'dogmatism, the moat that surrounds all bastions of classical ignorance, is characteristically categorical in its logical form' (1965/1979j: 295).

By contrast to categorical systems, Kelly offers a 'cross-referencing' or 'indexing' system of classification that has us thinking in terms of 'axes' that 'give the best theoretical structure to clinical observations' (1965/1979j: 300). There is perhaps a degree of prophecy here in the move in the *DSM-IV* to a multiaxial approach to classification, though some of the axes invoke some degree of categorisation within themselves.

In respect to this second dimension of concern with philosophical criticisms of clinical psychology, then, personal construct psychology does not fall to the critical responses to classification and categorisation. Indeed, it was making similar criticisms from the outset.

A caveat

William James (1907a, 1907b) long ago noted the limitations of psychology against the broader questions asked by philosophy, or what he referred to as 'metaphysics'. The distinction was in terms of philosophy being concerned with gaining insight into the world as a whole. One stepped out of this and into the special sciences – of which psychology was one important example – in order to make some advances by adopting various assumptions, assumptions which left psychology 'fragile and into which the waters of [philosophical] criticism leak at every joint' (James, 1907a: 467). Chaiklin (1992) asks, in passing, why a psychologist would bother entering into philosophical questions – there, as raised by postmodernism – concluding that the main value is ideological. Such questions force psychologists to examine what are the important problems of the discipline and what types of goals it should pursue. Wittgenstein is most pessimistic of all in noting: 'The confusion and barrenness of psychology is not to be explained by calling it a "young science"; its state is not comparable with physics, for example, in its begin-nings. . . . For in psychology there are experimental methods and *conceptual confusion'* (1953: 232e). He goes on to say that because we have experimental methods we believe that we have a way of solving problems in psychology; however, the methods 'pass the problems by'.

Given these observations, though not only because of them, it is of value to introduce a caveat into our discussion at this point. The simple aspect of this warning is that whatever integrity personal construct psychology might have in respect of the problems of philosophy, it remains nonetheless a psychology. It is concerned with our understanding of human psychic life, not with the traditional questions of philosophy. Indeed, this is recognised in various places in Kelly's writings where he differentiates his interests as a psychologist, and thereby what he is prepared to accept or assume about the world, and what the philosophers insist on; that is, the philosopher has more stringent criteria and demands.

In lodging our caveat we can look first to some general matters and then to Husserl's critique of *psychologism*. The point here is to simply remind ourselves of some territorial matters and to put in place a defence against a charge of finding 'the meaning of life and the universe' in what was intended from the start as a theory with but a limited focus and range of convenience.

As we noted, it has been epistemology that has both fascinated and offended modern philosophy. Since Descartes centred 'thinking' in human existence, matters built up to the point where by the mid-1970s even psychology had 'gone cognitive'. In these developments that centred episte-mology, it was logic that appeared as the core of philosophy. In the deliberations over logic, several terms have emerged to describe the different elements of what logic is dealing with: propositions, judgements and state-ments are the common ones and the relationship between them has been controversial. For present purposes, it is useful to highlight propositions and judgements.

In the debate over propositions and judgements, F.C.S. Schiller (1926) suggested that logic has been misguided by failing to make a distinction between *propositions* and *judgements*; in not seeing that truth has to be attributed differently or in a different sense to a proposition and a judgement. If in addition to a consideration of propositions and judgements the question of *meaning* was considered, and as a prior question, then

> it would have been seen that the meaning and truth of propositions and of judgments differ radically, and that difference splits Logic into two, which may be conveniently distinguished as the logic of verbal forms (or 'Formal Logic') and the logic of actual thinking (or 'psychologic').
>
> (Schiller, 1926: 338)

Schiller goes on to discuss how the meaning of a judgement, under 'psychologic', is *personal*; it is the meaning of the person who makes it. For this to be understood by another – well before he or she might want to discuss its truth or falsity – that other must be aware of the context in which the judgement was made, as well as a potentially unlimited range of other considerations; things like the speaker's motives, biography, problems and, perhaps more importantly, his or her purposes or ends. Of course, these matters are complex and controversial in philosophy itself. The proposition is sometimes identified with the judgement, and the problem of there being a difference between reality and our judgements and propositions about it remains.

Despite possible criticisms, these observations do drive home a need to take care in ascribing to an enterprise concerned with one level of consideration (how individuals actually go about their day to day business of making sense of their worlds) a level of consideration appropriate to another (ultimate truth, absolutes, logical relations). In simpler terms, we might say: that we think (or doubt, or reflect on things not available to or through the senses) may well be true and worthy of psychological study; but to conclude that we 'exist' by reason of this is a different question that cannot involve the type of activity engaged in by psychologists. Indeed, that last activity presumes existence. In simpler terms again, and illustrated from a different domain: to know good is not necessarily to do good; knowledge of good derives from logic and reason, whereas doing good in a particular case is a matter of individual or group psychology.

At this point we might recall that personal construct psychology is self-consciously concerned with judgements. A construct is a reference axis whereby judgements are made; that is, meanings placed on things or events in terms of our interest in expanding our understanding and the efficacy with which we operate in and on the world. The primary interest is to understand something of the world that confronts us, not to 'know' it in some philosophical sense. In like way, in everyday life we proceed as 'naive realists', prepared to make various assumptions about the world – that the floor will not collapse beneath me, that other people do in fact exist – while we await the philosophical resolution of the problems of the existence of the external world and our knowledge about it.

Kelly refers to the unlikelihood of philosophers being satisfied with the type of explanation utilised by the individual, including the individual acting as a psychologist, and how 'as psychologists, we have to get along with our human handicaps, and the limited knowledge we can glean about what follows what is enough to enable us to get along gratefully with whatever it is we are trying to do' (1966/1979k: 44). He notes that the question of whether a construct is 'logical or not has no bearing on its existence' (1958/1979a: 87). And he indicates that personal construct psychology is less concerned with the propositional speech with which logic deals, and more with psychological matters that concern not the 'single entity choice' of classical logic, but the 'double entity choice' of psychology. As he explains this, when a person says 'A is B' he or she is not only rejecting the alternative proposition 'A is not B', but also asserting that 'A is not C' (1961/1979c: 98).

In other terms, we might note that while the philosopher is adamant that the opposite of black is non-black (its logical opposite), we are more likely to live with it being white (its popular opposite). Even more significantly for personal construct psychology, however, is that we live quite comfortably with the opposite of black being 'happy' or 'Easter', or 'theatre', and so forth; whatever the philosopher says we are doing (il)logically when we make such judgements, we know psychologically what we are doing.

Rychlak (1996) has developed a more 'formal' notion of this sort of logic that attempts to accommodate some aspects of psychologic. Thus, if the opposite of black was 'Easter', say, this would be intelligible in a particular construct system because the 'logic of tautology', as he calls it, allows us to understand 'Easter' as part of an existing system of understanding. This might, for example, include constructs about the Resurrection and all it implies for a Christian.

Now, it may well be that both as an individual and a species we want our judgements to have the status of propositions and to be 'true'. However, as Rowe (1978) notes, there is no way of proving the meaning we ascribe to things or events; we are 'doomed' to the fact that the meanings we so ascribe may be ultimately meaningless. It is the task of philosophy to prove that they are not meaningless. It is the domain of meaning-making, meaning testing, striving for meaning – importantly, perhaps, meaning beyond the mere accidental or contingent 'here and now' – that personal construct psychology focuses on. In this focusing, it provides a most thoroughgoing account, as well as a methodology, but one concerned with meaning, not truth, with psychologic not logic.

A different focus for our caveat is Husserl's critique of *psychologism*. Traditional definitions of psychology mark out its territory as being concerned with the study of mental life. James (1907a), for example, saw it as the science of mental life, in terms of the phenomena of mental life and how these were dealt with in consciousness. In recent times something of a crisis has been identified in psychology as its methods, proper subject-matter and status as a science have come under scrutiny (Giorgi, 1981; Hillner, 1987). Hillner (1987) has identified the 'compositional problem' of psychology, its difficulty in saying just what it was as a discipline.

These internal debates aside, however, it is with Edmund Husserl that is articulated most forcefully the limit of psychology or, better, of *psychologism*. Husserl, amongst other things, set out to demonstrate that logic did not merely describe 'laws of thought' as existing in the mind and as features of the operation of mind, but rather described basic features of the world; logical relations were 'in the world', not established by the mind. Psychology could not be the fundamental science because it itself rested on more fundamental postulates. Husserl set out a critique of psychologism in his *Logical Investigations*, but a most succinct statement of the error of psychologism is given by Bolton:

[Husserl] made a distinction between natural and logical laws. The former are established through abstraction from the facts of experience and, therefore, can only be stated as probabilities. Thus if the psychology of thinking developed laws of thinking these would be natural laws and framed in terms of probable conjunctions. But there is nothing probabilistic about the laws of syllogistic reasoning, for example, where in a valid syllogism the conclusion follows with absolute certainty from the two premises. Furthermore, the validity of logical relations is not dependent upon the acts of judgement in which they are grasped; the empirical laws to which thought must conform in order to satisfy the ideal norms of logic are not the same as the norms themselves, and psychologism confuses this essential difference.

(1980: 248)

Husserl's initial quest, like Kant's, was to discover the pure essence of reality that lay behind or above everyday lived-experience which took that essence for granted. To do this, a special form of reflection was required, one in which the so-called natural attitude – the notion that reality consisted, ultimately, of a physical substance that was somehow 'out there' to be studied – was set aside. Thus, in the *epoché* or 'bracketing' of the natural attitude we suspend our acceptance of all that we otherwise impose on the phenomena of the world in order to catch consciousness in the very acts of imposing meaning on the world. This is well brought out by Jennings, who notes how

Husserl believed that phenomenology could 'ground' psychology by first performing the foundation task of clarifying the implicit preunderstandings and preconceptions of mental phenomena . . . .Basically, the forgotten distinction between phenomenology and psychology is that the former analyzes the essential character of various types of conscious acts, whereas the latter studies the empirical contents of actual subjective experiences corresponding to actual existent environmental events (i.e. subjectivized objects of the natural attitude).

(1986: 1240)

An example used by Jennings (1986) to illustrate the difference between a phenomenological and a psychological approach is as follows. This concerns the study of the impacts on a white community of a non-white family moving into their community. From the psychological perspective, one might study what 'colour' means to the neighbours and what constructions each places on the particular ethnicity in question. In his example, a psychologist might use a series of open-ended questions and perhaps a rating scale that measured racial prejudice. However, this would not constitute a phenomenological approach nor phenomenological data. Rather, the data collected deal with the facts of a particular experience. What phenomenology is interested in, by contrast, is not this particular experience of prejudice but the nature of prejudice itself, its 'essence'. As Jennings notes, 'The meaning-conferring act is an essence that transcends (i.e., is not relative to) historical age, culture, individual opinion, personal experience, and so on' (1986: 1238). The phenomenologist is interested in the universal essential way that, for example, an ancient Egyptian, Bronze Age hunter, a contemporary citizen of any particular nation, and so on, would construe a person of different race or ethnicity.

Given this difference in focus, however, personal construct psychology may perhaps offer something of a fully worked-out account of a level of the *operation* of consciousness that illuminates that grounding level that phenomenology is interested in. That is, personal construct psychology deals not only with the subjective experience of meaning-making, for example what something means to *me*, but adds two further dimensions: first, the dimension of the meaning-making process *per se* in terms of a system of constructs and a dynamic that sees us testing, validating, changing, bringing new elements in, and so forth; second, in its use of a standard – the world 'out there' – and the notion of validation, it avoids mere subjectivity and solipsism, and looks to at least the beginnings of shared meaning that may give the knowledge of essences that phenomenology seeks.

From the above example and this last response, it is clear that at one level personal construct psychology is concerned with mere subjective experience, and unashamedly so. Yet, at another, in providing a fully elaborated account of the meaning-making *process*, it offers a valuable perspective on the phenomenologist's own task. Moreover, in suggesting a view of humankind as an *inquirer* it perhaps provides a contribution to a philosophical anthropology, 'a philosophical study of the nature of man' which, though it 'may use psychology, neuropsychology, physical and social anthropology, sociology, it *is* none of these' (Greene, 1970: xiii). That is, personal construct psychology by reason of its particular approach goes beyond being a mere psychology.

As a final observation, we should not forget Piaget's (1965/1972) observations as a sort of caveat on our caveat. In the foregoing discussion we have been privileging philosophy by reviewing psychology against philosophy as some sort of superior activity. Piaget, however, reminds us that philosophy, too, has its illusions. He suggests that philosophy always works with the fruits of existing sciences (speculative and synthetic philosophy?) and that it had no special domain that science could not intrude into. More generally, philosophers are chided for believing that they have 'a right to speak on every question without making use of the methods of verification', and this is even more serious 'if they take the results of their reflections as a form of knowledge, and even as a higher form' (Piaget, 1965/1972: 215).

We might note the warning, then, that personal construct psychology is limited in its capacity to resolve, even to significantly address, the core questions of philosophy. Kelly (1955/1991) himself says as much when he asks whether his position is a philosophy or a psychology, and answers that it is a bit of both. However, it is, as he spells it out, more of a broadened psychology than a limited philosophy.

In general, philosophy is concerned with propositions concerning reality, psychology with judgements which concern meaning; so, too, with personal construct psychology.

Concluding comment

A number of issues or topics that are important in contemporary philosophical psychology have been considered in terms of advanced thinking about them. Such a consideration finds that personal construct psychology appears to assay quite well in respect of that thinking. Whether it be in philosophy of science, cognitive science, thinking about determinism and free will, or philosophical issues in clinical psychology, personal construct psychology would appear to have something illuminating to say and something which complements that advanced thinking.

In respect of philosophy of science, there is in personal construct psychology a position that keeps to the forefront the significance of the *human*. This recognises the value of differentiating the human from the natural sciences, at least in terms of what we hope to derive from our study, if not also methodologically. Developed in detail by Rychlak (1985), for example, such a focus situates personal construct psychology with an approach to studying human behaving that deemphasises *explanation* and reemphasises *understanding*. This places it in the tradition initiated by Dilthey and characterised later as *verstehen analysis*; an approach that looks to human intending, predicting, meaning-making. Personal construct psychology not only passively 'aligns' with this tradition, but it provides a method of accessing the individual understandings that the psychologist seeks to understand; psychology, that is, conceived of as our understanding of our own understanding.

In relation to cognitive science, there are various points of contact between live issues in that field and personal construct psychology. The legitimacy of discussion of mind and consciousness and the focus on subjectivity and on interpretation worry personal construct psychology not at all.

In respect to determinism and free will, an old debate in philosophy, personal construct psychology compromises the debate by recognising that we are both free and determined. We are free or determined always in respect of a particular field; never entirely free nor entirely determined. Moreover, within the 'field' that is one's construct system, there is a structural determinism in which higher-order constructs 'determine' the operation of lower-order ones.

Finally, in respect to clinical psychology, personal construct psychology appears to escape contemporary criticisms of the notion of 'mental illness', as well as criticisms of classificatory systems. From the outset, it has not found significant use for such a concept as mental illness, and has worked rather with what has recently been called for as a better focus generally; that is, on health and wellness, rather than illness. Thus the interest in optimal psychological functioning was prophetic for such an emphasis and consistent with the concerns that motivate it. Equally, Kelly's suspicion of classification and categorisation is more fundamental than merely being a quarrel with a particular system of classification. It was classification as categorisation that was rejected, opening up the possibility that is being more and more approached in recent times of classifying in terms of the notion of axes Kelly (1965/1979j) had talked about.

Across a number of live issues in philosophical psychology, then, personal construct psychology appears to find itself comfortably aligned with advanced thinking, or well placed to illuminate that thinking. However, it is well to remember our caveat that at the end of the day, no matter how exciting these alignments might be, we are dealing with a limited psychology whose project had but a modest aim.

7   Psychotechnology

Psychotechnology, applied psychology, technology

'Psychotechnology' refers to a so-called applied dimension of psychology. Bunge and Ardila (1987) find one significant origin of the term in the work of Edward Titchener (1861–1918), who argued that psychology, by which he meant basically laboratory study of the functioning of normal and abnormal mind, was to be distinguished from psychotechnology. This last was the application of knowledge gained in the laboratory to such fields as education, medicine, economics and the law. Actually, Titchener used the term *psychotechnics*, which referred to 'applied psychology' generally, and within this domain, medical psychology meant psychotherapeutics (1928: 33). Interestingly, James (1907b), in his lectures to teachers and parents, challenged that psychology, which was for him a science, had anything to say for education, which was an art: 'I say moreover, that you make a great, a very great mistake, if you think that psychology, being the science of the mind's laws, is something from which you can deduce definite programs and schemes of instruction for immediate schoolroom use' (1907b: 7); sciences never generate arts without the intervention of an inventive mind using its originality. More recently, the guiding image of psychology has become that of the 'scientist-practitioner', someone who combines scientific studies (though a particular style or conception of science; that is, positivistic, empirical, experimental) with practical skills. Kelly (1955/1991: I, 28/I, 20) was an early critic of such a too tight understanding of science, too extreme an understanding of Bridgman's (1927) *operationalism*. He likely would have had similar reservations about too freely translating Campbell's (1957) ideas in physics to the psychological realm as a way of legitimating quantification, and as strengthening thereby the claim to scientific status for psychology; though, again, a particular conception of science.

Here, we are concerned principally with clinical psychology and psychiatry. It is in the clinical sphere that personal construct psychology had its origins, has its 'range of convenience covering those events commonly covered by psychological theories but with a particular focus of convenience in the clinical area' (Kelly, 1955/1991: I, 185/I, 129). Interestingly in this respect, Bunge and Ardila make an observation that: 'It is possible that in the future the psychology of health, with its broad social and community orientation . . . will replace much of what is known today as psychiatry and clinical psychology' (1987: 252).

An interesting and illustrative perspective on these matters of psychotechnology before we go further is Erwin's (1978) discussion of behaviour therapy and its relation to behaviourism and behaviouristic learning theories. He argues that these three are conceptually distinct and logically unrelated, any relation that might be elucidated being merely historical. Behaviourism is a theory of mind, or at least a set of theses about the relation of mind and body or mind and brain. Behaviourist learning theory is a set of supposedly empirical laws or principles concerning how learning occurs (for example, laws of effect and practice, massed and spaced practice differentials in learning). Behaviour therapy is a set of practical techniques for changing behaviour. Erwin argues that behaviourism is false, behaviouristic learning theory rests on less than satisfactory empirical support, and neither can conceptually or empirically provide the foundation for behaviour therapy. Behaviour therapy developed from behaviouristic learning theory by assuming its version of how learning occurs, and by borrowing some of its terminology (conditioning, reinforcement, stimulus generalisation, extinction).

Now, this problem of therapeutic practice being adrift from alleged philosophical and empirical supports, identified by Erwin (1978) in the case of behaviour therapy, is not faced by personal construct psychology. Rather, personal construct psychology derives from practice and in a context of the theory's embeddedness in a more thoroughgoing philosophical tradition that itself centres practice, the lived-world. This is an important feature of personal construct psychology as 'applied psychology', and provokes the idea of personal construct psychotherapy as *praxis*, to be developed below. More generally, the problems Erwin discusses point up the value of a perspective on the human condition, such as personal construct psychology, having a sound nexus between its theory and practice, between the domains of philosophy and psychology.

Another preliminary matter is that while things may not be as bad as Wittgenstein (1953) had suggested, there do remain grounds for concern that we do not have much to 'apply'; despite, or perhaps because of, having much data but little theory to integrate it. We will come back to the notion of 'applied psychology' below, but suffice to note here the very real question of just what it is that we take it that we 'know' to 'apply'.

Finally, talk of psychotechnology raises a further question concerning technology in a more general way, and there has been something of an explosion of interest in technology among philosophers. Technology is conceptually interesting as well as quite significant for individual and group life. In fact, there is an established field, the philosophy of technology, which supports a substantial literature (see, for example, Bunge, 1976; Durbin, 1976;

Rapp, 1982) and a brief digression to consider some of the ideas expressed in that literature is of value.

A number of the writers in this field have drawn attention to the general impacts of technology in the domain of psychology. One of the seminal writers, Ellul (1954/1965, 1977/1980), for example, saw his task as 'awakening the sleeper', to alert us to the impacts of technology in our lives, impacts he felt we were blind to. Similarly, Marcuse (1941, 1955/1969, 1964/1970) has argued how the pressures of life in advanced technological society operate at the level of the unconscious and direct us into a 'one-dimensional' life where we no longer see contradictions and in which the individual is oblivious to the real state of affairs. Heidegger (1954/1977), too, was concerned with the capacity for modern technology to distract us from deeper questions of Being. Most generally, technology very effectively serves to immerse us in those 'particulars' of life – the everyday, relatively trivial cares, moods, concerns, ambitions, and so forth – that distract our attention from the more important questions. Of the two forms of thinking differentiated by Heidegger (1954/1968) – *calculative* and *meditative* thinking – the more important, *meditative thinking*, is lost under conditions of life governed by advanced technology. This last type of thinking concerns matters beyond the everyday and beyond that instrumentalism which is celebrated by technology. It highlights thinking as a 'way of living or dwelling' in the world that seeks a deeper understanding of the human predicament and of the nature of Being as such.

The term 'technology' itself is derived from the Greek term rendered as *techne*, and is discussed by Heidegger (1954/1977) as originally referring to a way of knowing. However, in modern times, *technology* comes to mean less a 'knowing' through practical encounter with the world, than a challenge to the world. Consistently with Ellul (1954/1965) in arguing a difference in kind not merely degree between past and modern technology, Heidegger (1954/1977) contrasts the windmill, which 'asked' of nature, with the dam, which demands of nature in blocking the river flow in order to provide primary power, on demand, for the hydro-electric power station.

All of the matters raised over the last half-century by critical theorists from widely different backgrounds and perspectives are complex and wide-ranging. Their 'bite' for a psychology of human beings is that they raise the question of whether psychology's pursuit of scientific status has seen the discipline play into the hands of the forces of technology that might be 'anti-human' (Tesconi and Morris, 1972). Koch expressed concern that the hope that the study of human *behaving* might become a science too quickly gave way to the assumption that it was one: 'The entire subsequent history of psychology can be seen as a ritualistic endeavour to emulate the forms of science in order to sustain the delusion that it already *is* a science' (Koch, 1973: 636).

Personal construct psychology and applied psychology

In respect to the matter of the 'application' of psychology, two problems present themselves at the outset. One concerns the contested nature of psychology as a discipline, the other the problem of what we might take to be actually 'known' from psychological inquiry sufficiently well enough to be 'applied'. This last incorporates questions of whether laboratory studies, and comparative studies of other animals than humans, can be generalised to the real world. It is not meant here to take issue with the whole of the psychological enterprise, and to conclude that there has been no advance in our knowledge of human functioning. However, this has been a strong theme of writing over the past quarter-century. Lewin's (1931) earlier concerns that advance in psychology would depend on moving away from an Aristotelian approach went generally unheeded, such that Henle (1986) a half-century later suggests that had psychology listened to Lewin it may not have 'gone wrong'. Kendler (1981: 309) described psychology as a science in conflict, recommending that the term *psychology* be replaced. More generally, Hillner (1987) has written of the 'compositional problem' in psychology, suggesting that it is impossible to provide even an unequivocal specification of what constitutes a psychological phenomenon.

Personal construct psychology presents an interesting perspective on psychotechnology. It does not lend itself to a lucrative test market or to 'gadgetry'. There is no standard test, no equivalent to the Rorschach, the MMPI, and so forth. When specific 'tests' are developed they are relatively inexpensive and easily duplicated. The Grid Test of Schizophrenic Thought Disorder, for example, which asks respondents to rate photographs in terms of provided dimensions such as 'mean' and 'kind' and 'happy', could use any set of photographs and the formulae and conceptual basis lie in the public domain (Bannister, Fransella and Agnew, 1971). Moreover, tests developed in areas outside the focus of convenience will be employed, but in terms of certain principles deriving from the theory itself and its focus of convenience. Psychological measurement will not have the function of 'fixing the position of the subject with respect to certain dimensions or coordinates – such as intelligence, extraversion, and so on – or to classify' as a clinical type (Kelly, 1955/1991: I, 203/I, 141). Rather it will be for the purpose of surveying the pathways along which the subject is free to move.

Now, before passing to our thesis concerning *praxis*, we might suggest that personal construct psychology returns the so-called applied dimension of psychology to something closer to the original meaning of the term *techne*. In personal construct psychotherapy, the intent is closer to the idea of working with nature rather than demanding of it. Psychotherapy's task is to 'enable the client, as well as the therapist, to utilise behaviour for asking important questions' (Kelly, 1965/1979i: 223). It is a psychological process of learning about the client's world in its widest sense, not imposing on that world. It is a 'psychological process which changes one's outlook on some aspects of life'

(Kelly, 1955/1991: I, 186/I, 130). More generally, personal construct psychology offers a distinctive way of approaching human relationships because of the particular way of viewing the individuals' relationship to the environment; essentially one of understanding rather than exploitation, at least psychologically. Most generally, psychotherapy is 'the orchestration of techniques and the utilization of relationships in the on-going process of living and profiting from experience that makes psychotherapy a contribution to human life' (Kelly, 1965/1979i: 223).

This said, however, Kelly (1966/1979l) warns against humanistic psychology becoming anti-technological. He notes that in his view it would be a mistake to abandon technology. Rather, the humanistic psychology he was expounding needed a technology to express its humanistic intentions. Thus, experimentation *per se* was not to be abandoned, merely a particular approach to it that objectified rather than *involved* the so-called subject of the experiment. When psychology's technology was mistaken for its theory, or, we might say, the goal embedded in psychology's project lost sight of in its methodology, or when the subject and the experimenter are understood as being different from each other, humanistic research was frustrated.

Bannister and Fransella (1971) differentiate personal construct psychotherapy from other approaches to therapy in similar terms to these last views. They suggest that from the point of view of personal construct psychology 'many current "psychotherapies" are better viewed as *techniques* rather than as total approaches in their own right' (1971: 132). This view is echoed by Winter (1988) in a most insightful paper that demarcates personal construct psychotherapy from psychodynamic and cognitive therapies specifically, with respect to sexual problems. In particular, he argues (1988: 81) that sex therapy suffers from a 'surfeit of techniques', and that personal construct psychotherapy provided an important underlying rationale for common practices deriving from different theoretical bases.

In respect of technology as a 'way of knowing', the methodology that is the various forms of repertory grid 'test' has as its aim the disclosure of aspects of the individual's way of understanding his or her world. Equally, the self-characterisation serves this same purpose of disclosure. More generally, the therapy situation itself is the basis for a scientific approach to an interaction, a cooperative venture that generates understandings. That venture involves a 'moment by moment' sensitivity to 'what emerges' from it (Kelly, 1963/1979f: 53).

Moreover, it is *change* not *adjustment* that is the aim of personal construct psychotherapy. Thus are overcome the objections of so-called radical psychology (Brown, 1973) which draw attention to the manner in which therapists too easily work with ideal and ideologically driven images of what a mentally healthy man or woman is. Those therapists then endeavour to make the individual fit this image, such that an anxious working mother might be induced to see her discomfort as arising from a choice of career over a (particular) image of motherhood, and urged to adjust to this image by giving up work. The aim of clinical psychology, as far as personal construct psychology was concerned, was neither diagnosis nor research, but 'the anticipation of actual and possible courses of events in a person's life' and any intervention was to bring about changes in a person's 'outlook on some aspect of life' (Kelly, 1955/1991: I, 186/I, 129–30).

Kelly (1963/1979g) challenges us with observations on clinical and applied psychology. He indicates that he has little time for applied psychology, and that is why clinical psychology is so important; and especially so is psychotherapy. His argument is that, like a view of humankind as stated in Genesis, the theories of the psychologists do not seem to hold up too well when we encounter real people in the real world. Adam and Eve should have been content and not transgressed; but they did. The laws of learning derived in the laboratory and attempts to derive laws from the study of individuals who conform are similarly doomed. This is not a plea to understand the general nature of humankind by studying 'abnormal' members of it; an issue once raised as a critique against Freud. Rather:

> I am not saying that the nature of man is the nature of the extraordinary man. What I am saying is that the nature of man is revealed in his extraordinary moments, moments that may be illuminated in the course of his psychotherapy.
>
> (1963/1979g: 214)

What he is rejecting here is the idea of 'application' as noted above, but less as a practical matter and more one of principle. That is, he is arguing that the issue is not one of whether we have anything to 'apply' by way of knowledge, but that we *cannot* have anything to apply if we work from the laboratory, and with 'normal' subjects, to the real world. Psychotherapy, though not only psychotherapy, provides an opportunity to see human beings in critical moments when conventional responses, expected behaviours, conformity to expectations escapes him or her and one is 'left with no resources other than [one's] own nature' (Kelly, 1963/1979g: 215). Clinical psychology becomes a 'focal and essential area and method of scientific inquiry' (Kelly, 1958/1979b: 226) in which the psychologist deals with the persons directly and in an honest, straightforward way. It works from the real worlds of individuals, from practice to theory; just as in personal construct psychology itself, 'theory followed practice . . . in somewhat the same way as "form follows function"' (Adams-Webber and Mancuso, 1983: 2).

Clinical psychology is thus conceived as 'pure science' (Kelly, 1964/1979h), a conception of client and therapist alike, and together, framing their interaction differently; that is, in terms of their verbs, in the 'invitational mood' rather than in the 'indicative mood' characteristic of the applied scientist. Clinical psychology as applied psychology attempts to *impose* this or that concept, law or principle – these concepts etc. are in any case but ways of construing what a particular psychologist finds important. Clinical psychology as pure science sees the client and therapist acting in the way of the scientist, framing hypotheses that challenge each of them. This is a process of dialogue, not 'banking'. Moreover, it is in the spirit of O'Hara's (1995: 301) exhortation to continue the search for 'noncoercive ways of arriving at shared meanings', a search which values the voyage more than the arrival.

Entrenched in some particular orthodoxy and interpreting 'for' the client, the therapist avoids challenging his or her own system of beliefs. The client is thus drilled to understand things the way the therapist does. Agreement is rewarded as the client having achieved 'insight', while disagreement is chastised and what he or she is doing labelled 'resistance'. Both terms, however, 'grow out of objective speech and the prestigeful use of the indicative mood in talking about psychological matters' (Kelly, 1964/1979h: 155). Personal construct therapy, then, is not the application of rules, laws or principles drawn from a body of knowledge, not the 'exploitation of "scientific findings"', but, rather, 'an application of basic scientific methodology' (Kelly, 1955/1991: I, 400/I, 297).

More interesting and radical in the present context is Kelly's (1964/1979h) challenge concerning 'applied psychology', for which he had little interest and for reasons central to his general theory. Rather, he raised clinical psychology to pride of place:

> An applied psychologist puts his verbs in the indicative mood, while the pure scientist uses the invitational mood. . . . But clinical psychology does not have to be an applied discipline. It can, in the very best sense, be truly scientific. . . . I do not mean that the clinical psychologist uses his clients as unwitting guinea pigs in an experiment . . . I mean that the clinical psychologist *can* be scientific in the therapy room, that the client *can* be – and indeed probably *is* – a colleague, and that the client and his therapist may come to talk to each other in the language of hypothesis.
>
> (Kelly, 1964/1979h: 154–5)

Thus, in a mode derived from the German philosopher Hans Vaihinger, Kelly (1964/1979h: 162) leads his reader through 'the language of hypothesis' and raises the challenge to regard clinical psychology 'as if' it were the purest of sciences. There is in this challenge a significant shift from questions of whether psychology has produced any knowledge, and whether the notion of 'application' has any sensible meaning, to a reconstruction and reordering of the psychotherapeutic relationship. In turn, it recalls Bunge and Ardila's (1987) assertion, but now with less discouragement, that clinical psychology would be replaced by the psychology of health. The rejection of applied psychology, as usually conceived, not only overcomes this prospect but offers a developed approach where the broad social and community approach Bunge and Ardila emphasise can be complemented by personal construct psychology 'in the field' and providing a methodology that advances understanding.

Elsewhere, Kelly (1963/1979g) argued a relationship between understanding persons and understanding the nature of personkind. We will go on to develop this point in connection with some later observations on philosophical anthropology, psychology, and personal construct psychology in particular. Here, however, we might note that in the exercise of working with the *potential* of individuals, and the limitations imposed on one achieving that potential, we gain insight into the deeper question of a human being's relationship to the real world which he or she inhabits.

Personal construct psychotherapy as *praxis*

These observations lead us to the suggestion that personal construct psychology as 'applied psychology' is a *praxis* rather than a *theory* or a *practice*. Let us pursue this idea a little further by considering the term *praxis*.

Aristotle distinguished between three basic forms of life or outlooks, only two of which were of real interest. One was the 'theoretical', understood as 'a particularly sublime way of life which was less shallow than that of mere pleasure-seekers and less hectic than that of "politicians"' (Lobkowicz, 1967: 7). The second was the 'practical', which was the life of politics but politics conceived in terms of honour and an idea of the Good. The life of those who equate the Good with pleasure, which was Aristotle's third category, was not worth consideration.

The term *theory*, in Aristotle, conveyed an earlier sense of someone who observed situations and events for the 'something more' that might be present in them, a life of observation, contemplation, reflection. It originated in humankind's awe and wonder, rather than from a need to solve practical problems, and it embraced what we now call science; at least, science as 'inquiry'. *Practice* is used of political activity, but, as Lobkowicz (1967) notes, it is not a clear term. It seemed to be used of various activities where some sort of general intent or outcome, as opposed to mere bodily labour, is involved; and, of course, activity other than reflection or contemplation. In each case, it was not a choice available to every person to follow either the theoretical or the practical, but one available only to members of the leisured class who were free from the daily tasks of survival. The debate within this class was, in essence, whether the contemplative life of the philosopher was superior to the active life of the politician. Aristotle's argument was that it *was* and had to be, and this because the contemplative life was further away from the level of day to day necessity than politics, and closer to our highest virtue.

The terms *theory* and *practice* were, then, narrowly located and ambiguous. With the shift initiated by Hegel, however, theory and practice are understood not as in opposition but the one in the service of the other. What we do 'practically' we do in order to advance contemplation: 'practice, taken as any action transforming a reality outside thought, is for the sake of theory' (Lobkowicz, 1967: 153).

Bernstein (1972) follows Lobkowicz in his delineation of *praxis*, drawing a connection with pragmatism. Having distinguished two senses of the term deriving from Aristotle, a 'high' and a 'low' sense, he relates the first to pragmatism. The low sense sees *praxis* identified with 'practice', whereas the high sense refers to activity in the social, political and ethical sphere of life which summarises to an idea of 'living well'. *Praxis*, in Aristotle and beyond, was linked to interaction in social and political life; life in the *polis*. The importance of the social-political context was, however, developed most forcefully by Marx.

Marx gave us the modern notion of *praxis*. However, as Lobkowicz (1967) reminds us, Marx used the actual term infrequently and in different senses. In essence, though, Marx reversed the direction previously noted; it was not from 'thought to action', but action, practical life, that generated thought. However, it was a particular type of activity and a particular type of thought or reflection. That is, *praxis* was any practice that 'results in a transformation of mind-independent realities which entails a humanization of man' (Lobkowicz, 1967: 419). It was the 'connection' between activity and the contemplation it originates that was what was important – as it had been in Hegel. But the connection envisaged by Hegel was stripped of its mystery in being tied up with the operation of Reason in history or the idea of Absolute Knowledge. *Praxis*, in Marx, was 'a central category of the philosophy which is not merely an interpretation of the world, but also a guide to its transformation' (Vázquez, 1966/1977).

The focus on that practice which enlarged our contemplation of what was truly human gave us the contemporary sense of *praxis* that is captured most fully in Paulo Freire's writings (Freire, 1972a, 1972b). Freire, too, gave us the related concept of *conscientisation*, which is also illuminating here. While Freire's writings had their own focus of convenience in the field of education, in particular in criticising 'banking' in contrast to 'dialogic' education, they translate very well to personal construct therapy. The idea of 'banking' education is that of a teacher who knows more and better, 'filling up' the ignorant student with information. By contrast, dialogic education involves a dialogue between two individuals who, as he says, 'make their Easter'. That is, each dies to old ways of thinking – for example, that one is naturally and always the teacher, the other naturally and always the pupil – and each is 'resurrected', reborn as a mutually curious human being.

Following Marx, Freire takes *praxis* as an inextricable interconnection of thought and action. The essence of the word *dialogue* is reflection and action in fundamental interaction. Reflection without action, action without reflection is not *praxis*. Words devoid of action are mere 'verbalisms'; action devoid of reflection is mere 'activism'. Real dialogue, *praxis* develops critical reflection and conscientisation, one of the more difficult concepts in Freire's writing.

The concept of conscientisation refers to a deepening of awareness to particular aspects of the relationships between people; in particular, to the 'situational' nature of all relationships: 'Human beings *are* because they *are* in a situation. And they *will be more* the more they not only critically reflect upon their existence but critically act upon it' (Freire, 1972b: 90). When reality, that is, the reality of the situation, becomes clearer, when dimensions of exploitation and oppression are exposed, the individual emerges from ignorance and powerlessness to awareness and a sense of efficacy. Thus emerges conscientisation, which is possible because while the consciousness of human beings is conditioned by social forces, the human being can recognise that it is so conditioned. Conscientisation is more than mere overcoming of 'false consciousness' and more than simply 'becoming aware' of the real nature of the situation in which one is immersed. It involves a critical insertion of the conscientised individual into a reality that has been demythologised (Freire, 1972b).

In a most appropriately titled piece, 'Knowledge, Action and Power', Matthews (1980) indicates that *praxis* presupposes realism; that is, an acceptance that there is a world independent of people. This world, moreover, is not merely 'catalogued' by the individual in a quest to know and understand it, but, rather, the comprehension we seek derives from our needs and interests: 'we come to know it in as much as it satisfies our needs and suits our interests' (Matthews, 1980: 85). Freire quotes Sartre with approval in connection with the problem of straying too far from the real world and thus into idealism: '"There are two ways to fall into idealism; the one consists of dissolving the real in subjectivity; the other in denying all real subjectivity in the interests of objectivity," says Sartre in *Search for a method*' (Freire, 1972a: 30, footnote).

Moreover, for Freire, the goal he stressed was to come to know the created world which expressed human subjectivity, and collective subjectivity (human culture), in order that we could recognise the impact of that created world on us; and thereby overcome that impact. In this, he stressed that activity that is education, and how 'learners must discover the reasons behind many of their attitudes toward cultural reality and thus confront cultural reality in a new way' (1972a: 35).

Now, this notion of *praxis*, especially as elaborated by Freire, appears a powerfully suggestive one for personal construct psychology as an 'applied psychology'. There is also strong circumstantial support for such an argument, given the significance of pragmatism for personal construct psychology, and of the idea of *praxis* for pragmatism. Moreover, at least conceptually, there is a response here to the concerns discussed by Neimeyer (1997) and Lutz (1997) that constructivist approaches to therapy are disingenuous, or at least naive, in regard to the real power differential between client and therapist. Some of this discussion might benefit from a differentiation between *power* and *authority*, but in principle, as Neimeyer, in particular, notes, there is 'nothing endemic to a constructivist model of therapy as conversation that requires a passive therapeutic stance' (1997: 59). Conceived as *praxis*, such therapy in fact takes on an inherently liberating stance. Moreover, it requires that the therapist him- or herself makes what Freire calls a 'political background choice' in favour of an egalitarian rather than an authoritarian outlook on the world. McWilliams (1988, 1996) has independently developed the relationship between the approach of personal construct psychology and the social philosophy of anarchism to capture the essential dimension of liberation that these observations here generally address.

There is also another speculative matter arising from Neimeyer's (1997) discussion of psychotherapy and connected with the idea of personal construct psychotherapy as *praxis* being suggested here. Neimeyer draws attention to the practical problems of working in therapy with a 'self' (both client and therapist self, presumably) conceived in some of the more nebulous ways self has been conceived by thinkers of the postmodern perspective. The *praxis* notion would presumably have less difficulty here, working as it does from practice to theory (contemplative understanding), from the real, live client in whatever 'guise' or in whatever mode of discourse she or he scatters her- or himself.

The therapeutic approach, eclectic as to method, has as its goal the elaboration of an individual's construct system in order to make it more 'realistic' *vis-à-vis* the situation in which the individual is operating. In its very essence, this process brings about an understanding that is satisfying to the individual, yet tested in action; that is, in behaviour. In turn, 'human behaviour makes the world a different kind of place – though not always a very good one to live in' (Kelly, 1966/1979k: 37). A passing reference to the concept of 'learning' is also interesting to the analogy with Freire being drawn here. Kelly (1963/1979f: 64) notes that what he is describing as psychotherapy could equally as well be called 'learning' as long as that term is understood as that activity which helps us get on with life.

Moreover, a state akin to Freire's conscientisation can be suggested as emerging. As Kelly notes of the person who has found therapy helpful: he or she 'often says, "In many ways things are the same as they were before, but how differently I see them!"' (1958/1979b: 227). A new awareness emerges that is the basis for new action in and on the world, just as conscientisation involves a critical consciousness that is not deluded by the 'givens' of situations. To be sure, Freire had in mind that a particular understanding would emerge; that is, that which saw the reality of exploitation, of inequality, of oppression. We cannot say that Kelly looked this far afield; indeed, his attitude to particular political or social ideas was either typically partisan for a citizen of North America (Holland, 1970, 1981) or sufficiently neutral to allow that 'anything goes'. In regard to his 'neutrality', Kelly's characterisation of the four major social-ethical systems – Judaism, Catholicism, Protestantism and Communism – in terms of their correspondence to four strategies for coping with the problem of good and evil – law, authority, conscience and purpose – is immediately self-censored with the observation that the matter is more complex. However, certainly personal construct psychology proposes a stepping off point for the type of change that Freire has in mind in its view of the human being as 'too recalcitrant to allow' circumstances to control him or her, and, as history shows, 'less and less disposed to accept the dictatorship of circumstances' (Kelly, 1966/1979k: 27). Thus, too, there appears to be here one productive, practical response to Gergen's (1992) call for a postmodern psychology that is emancipatory of mystifications imposed by social forces and interests.

Lest we become too enthusiastic, however, it is appropriate to recall Holland's (1981) observations at this point. Holland argued that *reflexivity* in personal construct psychology has to be taken with caution. He distinguishes a strong and a weak sense of reflexivity, the latter characteristic of personal construct psychology. Weak reflexivity is an awareness that one's own constructions, and one's own theories, are themselves products of humankind's attempt to make sense of the world. It is a matter of recognising that each of us has (merely) a different perspective, and that personal construct theory is but another perspective, one which grows up from our attempts, and humankind's attempts, to know the world. Strong reflexivity is exposing of ideology; it gets to the levels of meaning imposed by social structures and which are held not to be accessible to normal reflection.

This last charge has been considered in various places in the foregoing discussion and again returns us to the tensions between social and personal constructionist viewpoints. We do seem, however, to need individual minds to do the construing, to do the reflecting in the 'stronger' sense. Further, that ideology from which we suffer must not be so pervasive and all-encompassing as to be inescapable. That is, sociology of knowledge is possible because personal construction is possible and ideology can be, in principle, exposed. These are, of course, not new problems in social and political philosophy and the literature is voluminous in respect to Marxiology alone.

Despite the warning signalled by such commentators as Holland (1981) and Stefan (1977), and echoed in other assessments, personal construct psychology can be reassessed with advantage in terms of these matters of *praxis* and conscientisation. Just as with *praxis* in Marxism, the direction of flow of ideas is from the real lived-world of people to the 'theories' they form about their world and their life, and about Life. What Marx understands as consciousness, and personal construct psychology as a construct system, derives from the world of practice, broadly conceived. Equally, when the construct system is found not to be functioning, this is because of a mismatch between the social context and one's construction of it.

Concluding comment

The notion of a psychology being 'applied' to practical problems or problem situations preserves a particular understanding of psychology and therapy. While there are difficulties identified within psychology in terms of the promise of a scientific psychology not being fulfilled, of the generally limited state of our knowledge, of there being much data but little theory, personal construct psychology is again noted to raise a more fundamental difficulty. This is that the enterprise of psychology is flawed in its basic approach of trying to move from the laboratory to the world. As Bannister and Fransella (1971: 193) suggest, personal construct psychology insists that we experiment not *on* but rather *with* individuals. Thus might psychology be advanced in its understanding because 'two people struggling with major personal issues might prove a scientifically more rewarding focus for psychology than the navigational problems of the rat' (Bannister and Fransella, 1971: 124). In turn, psychotherapy is analogous to the relationship between a supervisor and research student, a partnership in which each struggles for enlightenment.

These observations accepted, a most apt way of conceptualising personal construct psychotherapy is in terms of the concept of *praxis*. It is not a matter of 'applying' a particular technique of therapeutic intervention, nor applying some law or principle established in some experimental situation. Rather, situations in which one person seeks help from another, like those where one person seeks to get to know another, involve 'conversations' or dialogue which is originative of understanding for each (Mair, 1970b). In that conscientisation which was for Freire the outcome of such dialogic encounters, there is a potent analogy for the image of therapeutic dialogue in personal construct psychology. As Bannister and Fransella put it in respect of psychology generally: 'The aim of the psychology of personal constructs, put at its most pious, is liberation through understanding' (1971: 201).

8 Political and social life

The focus of this chapter is the social-political dimensions of personal construct psychology, taking the social-political in its widest sense to include the broadest sphere of humans living together, and taking the issues within this domain philosophically, as indicated in Chapter 1. In addition to this general focus of the chapter, two other relevant matters are addressed: *ideology* and *religion*.

While the discussion here is not intended as a thesis in its own right, nor a particular contribution to social or political philosophy, two ideas stimulate the focus of concern and generate something of an argument or position. The first derives from a discussion in terms of 'historical psychology' and its attempt to place 'mind in nature' (Barbu, 1960, 1971). Historical psychology is concerned with the emotional climate generated by life in different types of society; emotional climate characterised by Barbu as a 'complex of feelings or a pattern of emotional dispositions and attitudes characteristic of a group of individuals in a given historical situation' (1960: 30). The second idea derives from a recognition of works which address the social and political ideas and implications of, for example, psychoanalysis (Fromm, 1942; Flugel, 1955; Roazen, 1968; Robinson, 1969) or behaviourism (Skinner, 1971; Hardison, 1972). The suggestion here is that personal construct psychology approaches psychology in the same grand fashion that allows it to be placed at least alongside these last positions as having a perspective on the general social-political conditions humankind constructs for itself.

The social-political in personal construct psychology

Personal construct psychology is relatively silent on political matters and this is in one sense understandable, in another somewhat surprising. The focus of convenience of personal construct psychology was clinical psychology and at least the pretensions of this discipline are to political neutrality. Yet, as radical psychology and in-depth study of the psychotherapeutic relationship suggested, there was more than a little to do with power going on in therapy, and more than a little about adjustment to the status quo.

Kelly (1962/1996: 40) ventures observations on the political scene in

Europe that represent his reflection on a 'once in a lifetime argosy', and of his own country through the eyes of others. The thrust of his observations concerned the overarching constructs that he identified in different countries as providing meaning for group life. These were conceived in terms of 'decision matrices', sets of dominant or overarching constructs that Kelly believed could be discerned in different countries he visited. Thus, in the Republic of Georgia, he found two of the most important constructs both socially and personally concerned *capitalism* and *education*. In the Scandinavian countries, even in the 1960s, he found a conception of North America characterised by cities, towns, and countryside of 'unbelievable squalor' and the 'abject hopelessness of the less privileged fourth of [the] population – of [people] living in despair, of dilapidated farms, of mental hospitals that look like mismanaged zoos, of fear and violence stalking' the city streets (Kelly, 1962/1996: 52). This is something of an open, objective report for someone who might otherwise have felt that his society and culture were being disparaged by such constructions.

Holland (1970) takes Kelly to task for some of his remarks about Europe and for his limited understanding of the theoretical position that was illuminating Russian efforts to rebuild after the 1917 Revolution. Significantly, it was historical and dialectical materialism that guided that rebuilding, and Holland felt that the theoretical positions that these expressions describe had much in common with the position which is articulated as personal construct psychology.

As suggested, politics is usefully construed as being concerned essentially about the distribution of power in a social system, and there are a number of discussions of *power* in personal construct terms, as well as in terms of personal construct psychology and psychotherapy. Kelly (1955/1991) himself had noted how power, force or energy constructs were commonly observed to be employed by individuals and how the proportion of these in a repertory grid might be of interest to an understanding of a particular individual. He was keen to remind us, however, that the acceptance of a power construct in an individual was 'not tantamount to embodying the notion of force in the psychology of personal constructs' (Kelly, 1955/1991: I, 240/I, 168). Interestingly, Scheer (1996) finds power within personal construct psychology's presentation of itself. Specifically, the English language in which the theory is stated and discussed effects a power differential that favours native English speakers. That is, there may be in evidence an example of 'Bernstein's two codes of speaking: the restricted and the elaborated code' (Scheer, 1996: 135). While Kelly cannot be blamed for this, Scheer's point is well taken, and the second generation of personal construct psychologists might need to consider how the position itself is articulated so as not to effect a behavioural contradiction.

There is nothing inherent in personal construct psychology to suggest any intentional favouring of the North American way of life, notwithstanding Kelly's (1962/1996: 33–4) possibly partisan observations on the Soviet Union.

However, as I have argued (Warren, 1996), there is an assumption of a flexible and open, crisis-free social organisation that is democracy that Kelly, perhaps following Dewey, assumes to be in operation. Indeed, such a system may be necessary for optimal psychological functioning.

Kalekin-Fishman (1995) argued that personal construct psychology was sensitive to issues of power in two ways, but perhaps too feeble in its effort to combat the misuse of power. One, a positive aspect, was in terms of the general empowerment that was proposed through therapy; the second was inherent in constructive alternativism: 'the power of the principle of constructive alternativism lies in its recognition that different people may be capable of adopting different stances of contestation at any given time' (Kalekin-Fishman, 1995: 30). The problem was its relative weakness in provoking larger-scale change in the direction of a better world; essentially the impotence of the theory for social reform. I have made a similar point regarding the notion of mental health (Warren, 1992a); that is, that there was too great a degree of neutrality in terms of the contexts in which a notion of mental health or, better, optimal psychological functioning (Epting and Amerikaner, 1980) or 'perspectivism' (Landfield, 1980) operates. The idea of perspectivism, for example, may need to be developed in terms of *content*, and in terms of a *social context*. Thus, I suggested there was value in developing the link to the type of thinking underpinning work on different 'mentalities'. This would move our thinking about mental health in personal construct psychology terms from an individualistic focus to a social-psychological one, but the last wedded to a particular type of outlook; that is, the democratic outlook (Barbu, 1956). Such a focus would not be uncomfortable for personal construct psychology.

Epting *et al.* (1996) remind us of concerns over the seeming individualism of personal construct theory and the need to recognise power differentials in real life. They argue that there is a dimension of personal choice involved in any situation, even when external circumstances are powerfully determining influences on us. Again, the perennial tension between changing the consciousness of people versus changing the material conditions under which they live is raised. These writers suggest that personal construct psychology would opt for the former; that is, a 'social revolution' as contrasted with a political one, in practical terms. They also draw on Rowe's observations concerning power being 'the right to define reality', the 'ability to get other people to accept your definition of reality' (1991: 28–9). While there are matters here to do with authority (*de jure* and *de facto*) as differentiated from power, and indeed authority as 'legitimate power', personal construct psychology does emphasise a role for both the individual and the social. It takes on board the real-life pressures *and* imperatives imposed by social life, and was never blind to the reality of those pressures. As Epting *et al.* note, echoing Sartre (1943/1966): 'While one cannot choose not to die, one can choose how to live.' Personal construct psychology is a way of dealing with the fact that a personal construct system operates in 'a way that allows for both personal constructions to be real and for there to be an external world to be reckoned with' (1996: 316).

Finally, more critically, Willutzki and Duda (1996) turn attention to what they see as an overemphasis in personal construct psychology on the 'power-holder', which poses the 'danger of reifying the power concept' (1996: 343). Their approach is avowedly social constructionist, and their intention to combine the individual freedom to construe with social and ethical imperatives. The focus, as with social constructionism generally, is on *interpsychic* processes, that is, the form and content of discourse between individuals. Their emphasis is on the relational or co-constructive aspects of power, power conceived as a communal construction and applicable to any interaction. The discussion here again raises the tension between personal and social constructionism previously considered and this need not attract our attention at this point. Two things, however, are of interest. First, Kelly (1955/1991) would not appear to be at all phased by the discussion, which is well accommodated by personal construct psychology. Recall Kelly's (1955/1991) own comments on how power or force may be employed by an individual and could be examined through the Repertory Grid Test, and notice the alignment of this with Willutzki and Duda's comment that 'any interaction can be constructed as a power-thematic, and any bringing up of the power topic can be denied' (1996: 344). Second, most of the rest of the Kalekin-Fishman and Walker (1996) volume is an elaboration of the social dimension of personal construct psychology and how, not only but particularly through the commonality and sociality corollaries, it accommodates social relations and shared meanings, even though the focus is primarily on *intrapsychic* processes. This is made most clear by Walker (1996), who sketches the type of disagreement between social and personal constructionists (or constructivists) we discussed earlier.

We have sampled here from papers that have directly addressed the matter of the social-political in personal construct psychology, and there are other relevant considerations of this in the Kalekin-Fishman and Walker (1996) volume. An interesting final observation on this idea of power is Rowe's (1996) view that to adopt a personal construct position is itself to become a threat to people in positions of power. She suggests that to allow that every person has his or her point of view that is prima facie valid and to be respected – which is a most democratic of viewpoints – conflicts with a view that there is an approved, 'true' view held by Church or State, and to which one must conform. An idea of authority or of someone being *in* authority in respect of some viewpoint or value clashes with such an outlook.

Elsewhere, Rowe (1991) concluded a discussion of power in terms of how personal construct psychology, with its emphasis on understanding, might sit in relation to Smail's (1987) assertion that most pathological emotional distress is a direct result of unequal forms of power. We can conclude this section with her observation:

If one is able to understand the processes whereby people become unable to realize their potentialities in public living, to learn how to make a bodily contribution to the social world, to treat each other with kindness and forbearance as ends rather than means, and to become, as it were, organic custodians of an unknowable future, the ability ethically to criticize the social structures in which we live is one activity to be preserved.

(Rowe, 1991: 212)

The egalitarian outlook

At this point we can move a little from the notion of power to its locus in a broader mental framework consistent with the understanding Rowe invites. In the previously mentioned Kalekin-Fishman and Walker (1996) volume I have argued the thesis that there is an implicit acceptance of, and at least a strong implicative connection with, a particular form of social organisation and political outlook underpinning individual construing (Warren, 1996). The argument was more focused in that last discussion which, as noted, combined with other arguments to combat the assertion that personal construct psychology did not have a significant interest in the social dimension of life. The relevant theme of that discussion for the present chapter is the focus on the 'egalitarian mentality'. This draws on work which directly addresses this outlook (Barbu, 1956), or work which focuses it 'by contrast'; that is, work on the opposing, 'authoritarian mentality' (Adorno *et al.*, 1950; Barbu, 1956; Rokeach, 1960). Each of these outlooks is intimately related to notions of power and authority, the second most obviously so; indeed, the essential core of the authoritarian personality is the dimension of submission–dominance.

It was suggested that both optimal psychological functioning and effective psychotherapy, as Kelly envisaged them, either require or imply a particular social context. Such a context is characterised by a high degree of freedom, by flexibility, by a tendency of members of that society to judge others as being of equal intrinsic worth to themselves and to display a non-exploitative attitude to other people and the world. This last context has been called *democratic*, and the outlook, 'mentality' or 'character structure' both emerging in it and necessary for its continuance has been identified as the *democratic mentality* (Barbu, 1956, 1971) or, more generally, *the egalitarian outlook*.

The egalitarian outlook is variously identified as arising with the ancient Greeks (Barbu, 1956), or with a new state of mind emerging only after the Renaissance (Fromm, 1942). It is fuelled, in turn, by the Reformation and the Age of Enlightenment, that Age now judged so harshly for its legacy of an idea of the individual, the 'subject' as the *I* which is aware of itself and delusionally thinks it is autonomous. That harsh critical judgement has been addressed elsewhere in this volume where we discussed its claim that 'subjectivity' was not a 'given' but was constructed, and constructed *only* or *significantly*, in and by language.

Egalitarianism, as real or an ideal in terms of these last developments, can be summarised in terms of it championing two beliefs: a belief that each of us should regard others as having equal worth and equal rights to ourselves; and a belief that others should be treated in a fashion that respects that worth and those rights. Kant's exhortation to always treat others as ends not means captures part of this idea. As a general social theory, egalitarianism is a normative position stressing equality of worth and regard, rights and freedom *from*. As a psychological outlook, it is characterised in terms of mental flexibility and the features of democratic mind offered by Barbu (1956); generally, a freedom *to*. These last features are a sense of being a separate individual; of being able to maintain a genuinely reflective, deliberative attitude, not a merely doctrinaire one; of being able to see things as they are rather than merely how you would like them to be; of living with a sense of ease, or leisure. Barbu summarises the 'democratic' personality, which is but the directly political face of the more general egalitarian mentality, as a type which shows sufficient flexibility in its inner organisation, attitudes, feelings, ideas and behaviour

> ... to understand other personalities as 'others' and not as its own projections, to co-operate and to construct a way of life on the basis of free exchange of experience with others; that type of personality which is flexible and free enough to avoid its rigid integration with the culture-pattern of its own group.
>
> (1956: 106)

Ideology

An important term in social and political philosophy, and one worth comment in the present context, is *ideology*. Although the term predates Marx's usage, he was to give it a fuller and richer meaning. Earlier usage of this term meant simply 'the science of ideas' (Williams, 1976), and this became broadened to give a hint of disapproval in terms of ideology signifying merely the theoretical or impractical. Marx (1845), however, gave the term its more powerful pejorative sense and also its 'psychological' dimension. For him, ideology referred to a 'false consciousness' in which an individual may think that he or she is acting with this or that idea in view, but in fact is acting in accord with another motive entirely; that other, real motive always residing in the dominance-submission relations of social class.

In Marx, then, ideology describes a mental state or set of ideas or beliefs that is illusory and which distorts reality. Ideology is a general tendency to represent particular interests – those of a dominant class, for example – as if those interests were the common interests, the interests of all individuals. Ideology can be described as a 'false consciousness' in that the misrepresentation is not conscious for the individual and the 'sufferer' remains unaware of the fact that particular interests, including even those that are not his or her own, are being advanced 'as if' they were rather universal and for the welfare and benefit of all.

Later Marxists, such as Althusser (1971), faced with the problems of the exact nature of the relationship between the 'economic base and the ideological superstructure', sought to split the superstructure into more and less determined levels *vis-à-vis* the base. This was to give some scope for reciprocity between base and superstructure, allowing one level of the superstructure greater autonomy and freedom from ideology than the other. However, while it continues to work with the base and superstructure notion, such a move imports the same logical problems with that notion. Further, in so far as it does allow reciprocity, it weakens the totalising of the impact of economic base on the superstructure, thereby weakening the Marxist account as such. This was a controversial issue within Marxist scholarship and points to some of the difficulties with this concept of ideology.

Nonetheless, a notion of ideology is helpful in understanding, for example, the manner in which individuals sincerely believe propaganda they are asked to propagate. To pick up again on the example of authoritarianism, someone of that style of personal construction might persecute a particular group because of a sincere belief that the interests of the race or of the whole of the rest of humankind are thereby advanced. In particular situations it will not always be easy to distinguish awareness that something is propaganda and the operation of ideology. Equally, it will be difficult to determine at what point what began as conscious, cynical propaganda changed into ideology as the propagandists are captured by their own propaganda. The notion of ideology is, then, not without value in social and political theory and comes into psychology chiefly through Freud, for whom unconscious motivation, rationalisation and displacement of motives was central.

Now, while an individual's wider construct system may not be immediately available and may need to be elaborated, there is no notion in personal construct psychology that that individual is somehow permanently blind to 'real motives' or the operation of different levels of construing, one somehow 'truer' than another. Rather, the very exercise of approaching the world, more particularly here the social world, as a scientist implies an outlook that would be open to the real nature of the forces and factors operating in that world.

Holland (1981) and Solas (1992) take a less sanguine view. Holland criticises personal construct psychology for its 'weak reflexivity', characterises it in terms of utilising a metaphor of knowledge that is overly individualistic, and identifies it as part of the ideology of 'liberal pluralism with the prospect of increasing consensus and harmony' (1981: 25). What is missing is a strong reflexivity which would allow exposure of the operation of ideologies, and he cites Stefan (1977) as exposing the weakness of personal construct psychology here. Stefan (1977: 284) had noted that the institutions which constitute our social environment are based historically upon systems of thought which in addition to any modest fostering of self-reflexive criticism operate more so as to prevent the individual from questioning the substance of his or her self-generated identity.

Holland (1981) suggests that this is one of the most succinct expressions of the operation of ideology which taints personal construct psychology, restricts its value, and, reading between the lines, exposes it as itself a product of ideology. If it was wedded to the insights of Marx and Freud, he argues, it would have greater potential for developing the strong sense of reflexivity. More particularly, personal construct psychology could benefit from the sociology of knowledge.

Solas (1992) also argues that there is an ideological dimension inherent in personal construct psychology. This has two interrelated aspects. One, akin to Holland's argument, is the manner in which language is treated more or less as benign in personal construct psychology. The other, directly related to the first, is the scant attention paid to the manner in which the individual is constructed by social forces which arise from conflict and a climate of exploitation. In ignoring this reality, personal construct psychology exposes its own status as ideological in expressing a 'false view' of the nature of the environment which is generative of the constructs that individuals use. Personal construct psychology is also said to perpetuate ideology by persisting with the notion of bipolarity; this is where, for Solas, deconstruction is an advance on personal construct psychology.

Two points are raised by these observations for matters presently under discussion. First, whereas critics from within social constructionist types of analyses usually have a fairly fixed framework of both analysis and 'moral imperatives' (for example, to end oppression, to supplant this for that form of social and political organisation), personal construct psychology is prima facie neutral; thereby of course, leaving it open to the charge of ideology and of supporting the status quo. That is, it does not proselytise any particular form of social organisation, but may thereby be conservative of the existing one: 'the absence of critical awareness of the ideological dimension of personal constructs perpetuates the reproduction of ideology' (Solas, 1992: 390).

One response to this view might turn around the problem with the notion of ideology itself; for example, the 'cheap shot' that every view but Marx's was tainted with ideology. Another might insist that personal construct psychology did *not* at all understand the individual as a 'separate, atomized entity', a view of the individual which appears to underpin arguments supporting the conclusion that personal construct psychology suffers from false consciousness (Solas, 1992: 390).

A second matter is that in so far as personal construct psychology does imply the types of values summarised as 'democracy' and 'egalitarianism', so, too, do the types of social constructionist analyses that might criticise personal construct psychology for its false consciousness. Moreover, in so far as Kelly expresses a *proscription* as much as a description in his theory (Walker, 1992), the values he implies would appear to be shared by the critics at least as a goal of life; that is, a broadened understanding through a stance of 'permanent inquiry' that itself exposes ideology.

In Tomkins' (1963) discussion of the idea of left and right as basic dimensions of ideology and personality, a middle way between left and right is suggested as the most difficult path. Indeed, Tomkins suggests that the 'middle of the road represents the most radical ideology rather than a compromise position' (1963: 398). The special difficulty lies in the fact that the middle way is made up of a creative synthesis of both left and right, whose perennial tensions generate two well-developed oppositions. For Tomkins (1963: 399), Kant, Beethoven and Whitehead represent such creative syntheses and this was one reason that they are seen as such significant figures in their fields, overcoming, as they do, both sides of the polarity. Kant 'unites the creative and subjective with the universal and objective'. In Beethoven, form 'never becomes an end in itself as in much classical music, and expression never completely overflows form and constraint as in much romanticism'. And Whitehead argues that a viable society is one in which tradition is combined with experimentation. Tomkins could perhaps have used Bertrand Russell's statement of the fundamental problem he was then addressing as an equally good example of the Whitehead synthesis: 'how can we combine that degree of individual initiative which is necessary for progress with that degree of social cohesion that is necessary for survival?' (Russell, 1949/1970: 11).

This middle way between left and right is accepting of change and reform, but not of the total dislodgement of thinking from past aspirations and traditions of thought. This would appear to accord more closely with the position of personal construct psychology, in so far as it can be identified with a position in respect of the tensions between left and right at all. In a similar fashion, the idea of 'permanent negation', which has been argued to be the essential characteristic of 'the left' (Kolakowski, 1957/1969), might without too much stretching be rather seen as characteristic of the middle way and of the type of mental operation going on in construing; that is, for example, in the full experience cycle. Someone not going through the complete cycle may, perhaps, be as usefully characterised as suffering from ideology as characterised as not functioning optimally. But a theory which itself focuses on such a cycle, and related processes, would be curiously labelled ideological. Clearly, these matters are more complex and suggestive for the wider debate between modernity and postmodernity; and the suggestion concerning 'permanent revolution' is itself most speculative. However, they signal caution at too ready an identification of personal construct psychology as ideological.

Personal construct psychology appears then neither to privilege a North American way of life – indeed appears realistic concerning the 'downside' of life in that society (Kelly, 1962/1996) – nor to be expressedly on the left or right as these are customarily conceived. It is reasonably taken as 'middle of the road' in terms of left and right as dimensions of ideology and personality, requiring an egalitarian outlook prevailing in the wider society for optimal psychological functioning to be possible. It is always pointing us to that creative synthesis of dichotomies, in the construction both of Life and of our own lives. In all of this it may be 'naive' in a real world of oppression and exploitation, but that is another question.

Religion

A powerful influence in human social and political affairs has been religion, and a final consideration of this chapter is an examination of its relation to personal construct psychology. I have examined this issue previously (Warren, 1993), and a brief review of those observations is pertinent before considering the matter in the social and political context that presently attracts us. The question arises as an interesting one because the essential idea that all constructions of the world are in the nature of hypotheses seems to clash with Kelly's own apparent commitment to Christianity. Fransella (1995) tells us that Kelly was reared as Presbyterian and knew his Bible well, using religious metaphors widely in his writing. She also draws on the first-hand experiences of several of his students who attest to his commitment. She notes Landfield's recall, however, that Kelly's religion was 'certainly not a literal kind of religion', and how Kelly may have seen religion and science as two ways of 'making sense of the universe' (Fransella, 1995: 22). There is surprisingly little by way of observation on the apparent tension between the theory and the man in respect of this question of religion. Fransella herself expresses it as a puzzle that Kelly was a practising Christian when this was not a particularly popular thing to be, someone who viewed both religion and science as creative processes.

The question of the relation between religion and science is an old one, answers ranging from a basic incompatibility of intents and outcomes, to a basic incommensurability of paradigms. Science, of course, has experienced a significant conceptual revolution in recent times, just as religion has changed in terms of the development of new religions or denominations within old ones. There is value in distinguishing the living element in science (essentially unfettered critical inquiry) from the formal aspects of science (what stands at a particular time as the methods or the particular problems addressed and these influenced by factors external to science). In turn, it is possible to see some value in distinguishing *doctrinal* religion from a more nebulous belief in a spiritual level of being. Nonetheless, it is most difficult to square the living aspect of science as critical inquiry with an acceptance of any particular doctrine. Lest this tension between science and religion be thought to represent a false dichotomy or a now outmoded point of issue, consider a recent observation by Hawking (1988). At the conclusion of a conference on cosmology in the Vatican in 1981, an audience with the Pope was arranged at which:

> He told us that it was all right to study the evolution of the universe after the big bang, but we should not inquire into the big bang itself because that was the moment of Creation and therefore the work of God. I was

glad then that he did not know the subject of the talk I had just given at the conference – the possibility that space-time was finite but had no boundary, which means that it had no beginning, no moment of Creation. I had no desire to share the fate of Galileo.

(Hawking, 1988: 122)

There was a personal construct psychology study by Todd (1988) which unintentionally highlights our present dilemma. He examined the meaning of religious belief in a sample of believers, disclosing the different aspects of what religious belief actually meant to different (Christian) believers. He suggested that if one's constructs of religious belief formed a constellation with few outside implications and was separated from superordinate constructs, then religious constructs had little importance to one's ultimate life concerns, and vice versa. He analysed two grids in detail, revealing marked difference between two Christian believers in what aspects of their beliefs they emphasised or most valued. Now, while this is all very well, and useful and interesting, it says nothing about ultimate truths, the veridicality of revelation, the reality of life after death, and so forth, which religions have traditionally argued about, and argued with science about. What and how a believer construes is removed from the truth claims of religion or particular religions.

From a more social and political point of view in relation to religion, matters are often less friendly. Marx saw religion as a kind of anaesthetic which numbed the proletariat to the reality of their oppression in this life with the promise of a better life to come. Bertrand Russell (1927/1996) argued that religion was based on *fear*, promoted ignorance and subservience. Further, an argument can be made out that the idea of the holy posited by Otto (1923), or the 'courage to be' theorised about by Tillich (1952), grows from an under-lying dynamic that expresses a 'fear of freedom', a submissiveness, and, given the right social conditions, an eventual authoritarianism.

This last type of thinking, which finds religion restrictive rather than expansive for individual and group life, generates the issue of whether a model of the person as scientist, that is, as critical inquirer, can allow a commitment to an area of belief that makes knowledge claims that are beyond *substantive* critical inquiry. The matter turns on the manner in which the scientist goes about his or her work, basing theories on observable, tested, publicly available facts, and rational arguments, in contrast to the religious appeal to unseen, sometimes private experiences that could not be scrutinised in anything like a public, objective fashion.

Personal construct theory would seem to relativise religion. Religion is seen as just another set of beliefs and experiences, construed by different individuals differently. The psychology of religion would then be an appropriate field of inquiry that attempted to uncover different meanings of religious belief in individuals and groups. This meaning may stem from any one of the common dimensions of religiosity: theism, fundamentalism, ritual, mystical, church orientation, altruism, idealism or superstition (Maranell, 1974). Or, it may be the outcome of fear or a 'fear of freedom' that issues in the general down-grading of the individual and a vilification of the *human* in the face of a belief in something *superhuman*.

These psychological aspects of religion are not what most religions claim to illuminate. Most religions claim *truth*, something beyond mere personal individual belief and independent of, or tangential to, one's upbringing, life experiences, biography, and so forth. Personal construct theory, by contrast, appears to call for an atheism or at least an agnosticism in relation to organised religion. Religious *belief*, or the acceptance of doctrine, must signal on the personal level what Kelly (1965/1979j: 294) in a different context calls a 'hardening of the categories'. On the epistemological level it must signal an absolutism that is inconsistent with the openness underpinning personal construct theory.

This, then, appears to be a problem, but in a previous visit to it a number of ways forward were suggested (Warren, 1993). One of those suggestions was in terms of developing a view of religion that brought it closer to the social-political domain and which followed the social thought of Hegel. Thus might we offer a reflection on Fransella's (1995) question as to whether Kelly might have been thinking along the lines of developing or extending Christianity in terms of his thinking that grew into personal construct psychology.

As noted in our survey of philosophy, Hegel broke with the dominant theme of the so called 'Christian Centuries' (Payne, 1967) which saw western philosophy concentrated in and on matters *theological* and *religious*. Hegel found this concentration had not produced any advance in understanding and suggested that questions concerning the truth value of religious statements and claims were too difficult to answer and that agreement on them was unlikely. It was more fruitful, he argued, to examine what were the effects or consequences of people holding religious beliefs, acting as if their beliefs were true and the beliefs of others untrue. On his analysis, the consequences were *divisiveness* and the separation of people into antagonistic 'in' and 'out' groups. This was expressed in his notion of *alienation*, which the young Marx was to find so attractive; alienation of person from person, of the individual from his or her powers of understanding and labour.

However, Hegel found that this divisiveness and alienation was not observed in the operation of the ancient Greek folk religions. Moreover, it was not true of the 'real' message of Jesus, as distinct from the interpretations of that message by the Church. Greek folk religions *harmonised* Greek society and the different aspects of individual mental life (emotions, thoughts and behaviour); rather than dividing it or alienating its members from each other or from the different elements of themselves. Equally, Jesus taught an ethic of *love* which the Church perverted into an ethic of *authority*; from a focus on what one might do naturally to a focus on those who know better and command or manipulate obedience. In respect of Christianity, Hegel analysed how and why Jesus' teaching became distorted.

Hegel had initially been attracted to the Kantian moral position but came to consider this as mistaken because it still placed the basis of morality in the *commands* of others. In one way or another, either externally through threats and punishment or internally through the internalisation of specific commands as in what was to become a notion of 'conscience', particular behaviour was regarded as 'good' and *had* to be followed; there was a duty to follow it. Thus was the Sermon on the Mount understood. Jesus was assumed to be emphasising a proper 'reverence for the laws', which laws had to be followed if one was to do one's duty and act rightly. Hegel argued, however, that certain emotions, outlooks, inclinations, and so forth, were *naturally* good. He developed this idea through an examination of the notion of *love*; love was an emotion which led one to do naturally, without command, what *would have* been commanded as good, should a command have been necessary:

> The Sermon does not teach reverence for the laws; on the contrary, it exhibits that which fulfils the law but annuls it as law and so is something higher than obedience to law and makes law superfluous.
>
> (Hegel, 1798–9/1961: 212)

Hegel went on to develop the notion of *Sittlichkeit* (the *ethical* life) as contrasted with *Moralität* (morality, moral rules). These were psychological concepts that characterised states of mind; a *free* (autonomous) contrasted with an *unfree* (enslaved) state of mind, respectively. The 'good' was identified with the state of mind or a 'way of going on' of mind, that did not need to be commanded, nor to seek to command others. This can be better understood in terms of *egalitarianism* or the egalitarian frame of mind which we have earlier contrasted with an authoritarian frame of mind. For Hegel, we will find goodness to be a quality of mind, initially captured in the concept of *love*, this developing, as he saw the wider ramifications, into the notion of the 'ethical life' that we might recognise in an egalitarian outlook.

These ideas find later expression in social-political theories such as anarchism and in the rediscovered libertarian strand in Marxism that was expressed in at least some elements of the New Left. Some of the early anarchists claimed Jesus as a forerunner of their own views and one contributory theme to that theory was the affront articulated especially by the Anabaptists at any authority being accepted over human beings other than God's authority (Woodcock, 1986). Less religiously, one of the better and better known anarchist theorists, Peter Kropotkin (1902), stressed the general importance of any species working with rather than against its kind, and the human capacity for cooperation and mutual aid that is as often and more constructively manifest in human history than competitiveness and aggression. Such capacities alert us to a significant and very basic level of *commonality* and *sociality* in our individual constructions of the world, and the function of these capacities in promoting social cohesion. Moreover, there is here a return to the notion of *community* that Rousseau had promoted. The type of factors operating in a life in community go to more deeply human aspects than life in 'society', where we are seen by Rousseau as mere social atoms united but for instrumental purposes and where our natural capacities are perverted.

The antagonism between science and religion continues despite efforts to reduce the significance of science in human affairs, at the very same time as some religions claim the status of science; the creation–science debate is a case in point. This antagonism would appear to pose a special problem for a theory which takes as its model 'man the scientist', yet looks sympathetically on religion. However, if religion is understood in terms of an outlook of mind characterised in terms developed from Hegel as the egalitarian outlook that expresses his concept of *love*, then there may be some degree of minimisation of the problem – if it is a problem – within personal construct theory. This is an approach of rediscovering the essential nature of religion as the progressive unfolding of 'love', the 'ethical life', as a more general principle of uncoerced, free, spontaneous social life.

This is one way forward and it would not appeal to those who want a more objective and transcendental perspective in relation to religion. If this last perspective is to be defended, however, the onus would appear to lie with such proponents to indicate how such a wish could avoid offending the model of the person as a scientist.

Concluding comment

We have explored the connection between the domain of the social and political, and personal construct psychology. The suggestion has been that it appears either to be neutral to particular social-political orientations (neither right nor left), or to assume a democratic social-political system – or at least a system that encourages the egalitarian outlook – as underpinning at least optimal psychological functioning. In respect of the first alternative, it is perhaps particularly vulnerable to attack from both sides of the left–right spectrum which would claim that neutrality was impossible. In respect of the second, it is in danger of being dismissed as 'ideological' and as merely perpetuating a particular social-political system.

If the democracy to which personal construct psychology appeals is understood in terms of a frame of mind or mental outlook the way Hegel and Spinoza, and later Barbu, so conceive it, then the first attack is misplaced. Democracy conceived in this way, as but a specific appearance of a more general egalitarian outlook, favours no particular current political regime. Indeed, the critical voices of political philosophy of recent times, such as Herbert Marcuse, were themselves attacked as much by the left as by the right, by institutions perpetuating North American values as much as by those concerned with Soviet interests.

As to the second alternative, that is, the charge of ideology, personal construct psychology is again in an analogous position to the early critics of

Marx, critics whose ideas grew into the existentialist response (Carroll, 1974). That is, in their belief that by merely exposing ideologies we can begin to overcome them, these thinkers, like personal construct psychology, are themselves condemned as ideological. Rather, the real task was action, for, as Marx (1845) says in his 'Eleventh Thesis on Feuerbach': the philosophers have only interpreted the world, the point is to change it. Still, the argument continues as to whether a change in thinking has to precede a structural change, or vice versa, with equally vigorous support available for each side. Further, however, from another perspective, it might be asked just where psychology and psychotherapy stop, and political action starts.

The personal construct psychology perspective on religion can be developed in a similar way to the understanding of democracy. Religion conceived in the way Hegel was suggesting may provide an understanding of Kelly's own religious commitment and how this harmonises with the theory he developed. In essence, in terms of the present chapter, this issues in an ethic of love as opposed to an ethic of authority and power, which, in turn, has implications for social and political thinking. All of these matters are open ones and all of the areas of concern to philosophy of the social and political domains are ones where personal construct psychology has least to say in specific terms. Nonetheless, we have hopefully presented here at least a provocative construal of personal construct psychology in the social-political context.

9   Being human, making meaning

From all of the foregoing discussion it can be suggested that personal construct psychology is a substantive position in psychology, enlarging our understanding of human psychological and social-psychological functioning. This might be argued from its comprehensiveness as a theory, even despite or perhaps because of the flexibility of interpretation to which it lends itself (John and Soyland, 1990). It might be argued from the range of matters in philosophy for which it has something to say, or which, in turn, enlarge rather than disown its own outlook. It might also be argued from its concern with meaning that is more than merely subjective meaning. That is, the meaning to which individuals aspire is more than that which pertains at the mundane level of life. Human beings appear to aspire to 'higher' levels of meaning, meaning not only *in* life but also *of* life, and of Life.

There is an interesting complementarity in respect to this last point between personal construct psychology and the work of Viktor Frankl (1962, 1967), though one that has not generally been taken up by commentators. Frankl survived some of the most destructive of life conditions of modern times to reflect on the psychological temper of those who did so, identifying the significance of recognising oneself in terms of the totality or wholeness of Life. From this reflection he formed a theory based on three interconnected principles: freedom of will, will to meaning, and meaning of Life. Frankl sees meaning not as something we are 'driven' to, nor as something we 'need' – it would, as either of these, be but a means to other ends – but as a core aspect of our being. The Freudian view, which, for him, in particular focuses on drives and needs, sacrifices 'the fundamental fact which lends itself to a phenomenological analysis – namely, that [the human being] is a being encountering other beings and reaching out for meanings to fulfil' (Frankl, 1967: 19). In one of his oft-quoted anecdotes, Frankl describes how a patient depressed over the death of his wife was asked how she might have felt had he died first. The reply that she would have suffered terribly led to a reconstrual of the patient's own feelings and relief from his suffering because he 'suddenly saw his plight in a new light, and re-evaluated his suffering in the meaningful terms of a sacrifice for the sake of his wife' (1967: 26).

It is this level of construing that Rowe (1982, 1991) has consistently drawn attention to in her articulation of the core principles of personal construct psychology. Thus, she refers to our discovery of the axioms of life which establish rules and beliefs that link our constructions of ourselves to a place in the scheme of things and our futurity (Rowe, 1982). Our failure to accept the fragility of all and any of those axioms of life pushes us further away from fulfilment (Rowe, 1991). Moreover, echoing Frankl, she argues how 'when we reduce our life to nothing but meeting our physical needs and acquiring money and possessions we create a life which demeans us' (1991: 342).

Now, when the meaning to which individuals aspire is taken at this supra-individual level there is in place a task akin to that which Dewey identifies of philosophy itself. For Dewey, philosophy was 'a form of thinking, which, like all thinking, finds its origin in what is uncertain in the subject matter of experience, which aims to locate the nature of perplexity and to frame hypotheses for its clearing up to be tested in action' (1916/1966: 331). Indeed, such was also one aspect of Husserl's (1954/1965) conception of the origins of philosophy and the domain of its proper, though lost, operation. When early human beings shifted from the reflection on facts – everyday aspects of their everyday lives – to ideas, they were transformed:

> With the first conception of ideas man gradually becomes a new man. . . . This movement from the very beginning involves communication and awakens a new style of personal existence in its vital circle by a better understanding of a correspondingly new becoming. In this movement first of all (and subsequently even beyond it) a special type of humanity spreads out, living in finitude but oriented toward poles of infinity. By the very same token there grows up a new mode of sociality and a new form of enduring society, whose spiritual [mental, intellectual] life, cemented together by a common love of and creation of ideas and by the setting of ideal norms for life, carries within itself a horizon of infinity for the future – an infinity of generations finding constant spiritual [mental, intellectual] renewal in ideas.
>
> (Husserl, 1954/1965: 160)

Husserl goes on to examine in more detail the origin of 'philosophical and scientific man' and how the European world view has centred in it a spirit of philosophy as concerned with 'reason'. Thus, the crisis to which he alerts us is a crisis of *rationalism*. However, 'the reason for the downfall of a rational culture does not lie in the essence of rationalism itself but only in its exteriorization, its absorption in "naturalism" and "objectivism"' (Husserl, 1954/1965: 191). The significance of his point is made clearer here if we recall the distinction between reason and intelligence that Fromm (1956/1968) had reiterated. Reason was our faculty for *grasping* the world by thought; intelligence our ability to *manipulate* the world. Reason searched for the truth and was an essentially human quality; intelligence belonged to the animal part of humankind.

In this context of the recurrent theme of personal construct psychology being centrally concerned with our meaning-making, we are quickly brought into that development in philosophy that is *hermeneutics*. A discussion of the development of this approach in philosophy is illuminating for our theme and helps to elaborate personal construct psychology in terms of this tradition.

Hermeneutics

Hermeneutics was known at the time when personal construct psychology was gestating and also when it was being given its formulation, and known in even its modern form. Indeed, while they appear to have been significantly unknown to each other, the work of the Continental phenomenologists was in parallel in many respects to American pragmatism, particularly the work of Peirce. Hermeneutics had, however, an interesting history as a mode of doing philosophy, and this is usefully recalled by way of a sketch of just what this perspective is about.

Friedrich Schleiermacher (1768–1834) had extended hermeneutics from being a set of rules for interpreting biblical texts to a more thoroughgoing approach that took into account two aspects or dimensions of any act of speech or writing. One was what he called the *grammatical* aspect; the other the 'technical' or *psychological* aspect. The first referred to the rules that a speaker or writer is following, and these are bedded in the total speech activity of a time and place. The individual speaker or writer is here merely a 'location' or 'coagulation' of language as a broader social force. The psychological dimension recognised that in the individual's life the use of language and writing is one moment in the individual's 'biography'. The words chosen, the manner of their use, the context in which they are used, and the feelings aroused in and by that language are as important to the complete understanding of a particular text as is a thorough knowledge of the language itself.

As the theologian Karl Barth notes in commenting on Schleiermacher's concept of hermeneutics, for the adequate study of biblical texts, for example, what was required was *both* types of interpretation: 'an integration of the two approaches, the grammatical and the psychological; an integration so close that a text cannot be understood psychologically unless it is also understood grammatically and vice versa' (1923–4/1982: 180). Nonetheless, sometimes a more grammatical understanding might be to the fore, at other times a more psychological one, according to the topic being studied: 'Purely historical texts, for example, demand a minimum of psychological interpretation and letters a maximum' (1923–4/1982: 180). However, for Schleiermacher we can never achieve a final understanding of the psychological dimension and that goal is only ever approximated: 'There are still conflicts over Homer. . . . Not only do we never understand an individual view exhaustively, but what we do understand is always subject to correction' (1977: 149).

In any event, the postmodernist distrust of Schleiermacher's hermeneutics is misplaced. The contribution of that hermeneutics is that rather than being lopsidedly psychological its unique contribution is not the psychological nor the grammatical interpretation, but hermeneutics as 'an artful movement between the two' (Huang, 1996: 252).

Dilthey (1976), who wrote a biography of Schleiermacher, published his influential paper distinguishing 'explanation' and 'understanding', and this moved hermeneutics further toward its modern form. The interpretation of texts through the expanded notion of hermeneutics generated by Schleiermacher was extended to the whole of human history. Thus texts, documents, letters, statues, monuments, and so forth, represented the solidified form of life in past ages, and hermeneutics was conceived as a method of interpreting these. Through this hermeneutic interpretation we came to understand past life and our own, and the continuities that constitute a cycle of life. For Dilthey, in the study of these things of the past, a different type of outcome was called for than applied in the study of natural phenomena and events. This was *understanding* rather than *explanation*.

While Dilthey had made a distinction between methods appropriate to the study of 'matter' and those appropriate to the study of 'mind', when we turn our attention to the study of human beings these methods had to be combined. Mind and matter were but convenient concepts abstracted from experience and to be approached via different methods. However, when attention was turned to the human being as a psycho-physical unit, both approaches were required. Thus, Dilthey's theoretical framework can accommodate any kind of approach from ethnomethodology to physiological psychology (Rickman, 1976: 12). In another direction, Mead (1948) advanced the pragmatic consequences of Dilthey's notion of the 'inner life', focusing more on action, and there are to be noted generally 'important similarities in the systematic architecture of both hermeneutics and pragmatism' (Jung, 1995: 662).

The search for understanding is a basic feature of human being and of human interaction, emphasised particularly in the significance of *encounter*, that is, a 'recognition of the I in the Thou' (Dilthey, 1976: 298). Thus, as Rickman (1976) summarises it, Dilthey argues that the mind has an innate structure which generates the typical relations between perceptions, memories, needs and actions; mental life is purposive; individuals are aware of the two-way relation between their actions and the environment; mental states are expressed intentionally and unintentionally in physical states of the organism; and the world is not just perceived but evaluated in terms of feelings that it engenders and the impact of it on our purposes.

Heidegger came to hermeneutics and challenged what he saw as Dilthey's overstress on 'method'. For Heidegger, hermeneutics was not a method of approaching the world but the very essence of 'the original attitude towards the peculiar structure of the Dasein' (Bubner, 1981: 29). Heidegger transformed Husserl's original phenomenology into hermeneutics as an *ontological* position. He takes the original Greek words *phainomenon* and *logos*, words that compounded make *phenomenology*, and looks to their original significance. Amongst other meanings, the first means 'that which shows itself forth', and the second, judgement of 'that which lets itself be seen'. Thus, Heidegger (1927/1978) frames the human task as that of reading off the meaning of consciousness itself – of Being in its essence, or ontologically – by reference to the 'text' that was 'being in the world'. The inescapable, *ontological given* is our thrownness into a world we must interpret and understand: 'the phenomenology of Dasein [being-in-the-World] is a *hermeneutic* in the primordial signification of this word, where it designates this business of interpreting' (1927/1978: 62).

And why must we interpret or reflect? Because our existential reality is that of reflection, a reality we can be distracted from but which comes back rapidly when we have thrust to the forefront of our consciousness the reality of our limited existence in the fact of our inevitable death, our *non*-being. This last was Heidegger's account of the impetus for original reflection. Kierkegaard had another, similar, account in terms of the 'solemnity of the encounter with the nothing, which found confirmation in real historical catastrophes' (Bubner, 1981: 39). And Husserl found the impetus for reflection in the impact of the outcomes emerging from scientific activity that had drifted too far from the ordinary worlds of ordinary people. This generated a 'crisis' which was experienced as a loss of certainty, meaning and direction that, in turn, encouraged philosophical, that is to say, fundamental, reflection.

Now, Bernstein (1983) suggested how the confluence of various developments in relation to how human rationality was viewed led us 'beyond objectivism and relativism'. He saw developments in hermeneutics providing a view of human life that finds deepened understanding in the recognition of the centrality of our life in 'community', in dialogue. This leads to a recovery of the hermeneutical dimension of science, particularly for us in psychology, in the social or human sciences: the *Geisteswissenschaften*. Yet, this was more than a 'turn' in history of these matters, and in the philosophers who initiate and develop it in its strongest sense (Heidegger and Gadamer) hermeneutics concerns a fundamental ontological given, that is, our will to understand. We are each 'thrown' into the world as creatures who inescapably strive to understand and interpret, and 'if we are to understand what it is to be human beings, we must seek to understand understanding itself, in its rich, full, and complex dimensions' (Bernstein, 1983: 113).

Bernstein (1983) was elaborating the ideas of Gadamer, whose views are finally pertinent to the historical developments being sketched here. Gadamer (1960/1975) took Heidegger's hermeneutics and saw it as illuminating the common grounding of all of the specialised attempts to glean knowledge of and from the world. In the spirit of Husserl, Gadamer's hermeneutics was an attempt to understand the underlying principles that guide all the sciences and to expose deeper dimensions of the questions posed by these specialised sciences. These dimensions will illuminate the fact that all of the alleged divisions within and between the sciences, between 'nomothetic' and 'idiographic' or between 'explanation' and 'understanding', are still secondary to a deeper level at which the human sciences share a search for understanding. 'The phenomenon of understanding not only pervades all human relations to the world. It also has an independent validity within science and resists any attempt to change it into a method of science' (Gadamer, 1960/1975: xii). Further, the most basic and encompassing medium for this understanding is the 'irreducibly *linguistic* character of our relations to the world and to human beings' (Bubner, 1981: 56).

Gadamer outlines a position which sees our locatedness in linguistic structures nonetheless leaving an avenue for escape from them. This occurs through dialogue, genuine dialogue, with others in which the parties speak from different positions even within a common locatedness.

In this last development were to emerge new controversies for hermeneutics in a time when, by implication from Gadamer's work, 'philosophy itself can no longer be anything but hermeneutical' (Page, 1991: 127). As Block notes, just as modernism and structuralism were followed by postmodernism and poststructuralism, so 'an even older critical tradition, hermeneutics, has now been followed in its turn by a post-hermeneutical movement' (1991: 269). Significantly illustrative is Caputo (1987), who develops a *radical hermeneutics*, based on an insistence that we recognise the reality of the ultimate 'flux' of everything that is. However, as is the way of things, Block (1991) takes issue with Caputo, suggesting a more widely applicable criticism that in the end, despite all the stress on 'flux', Caputo, like other deconstructionists, frames ideas of a stable world: 'deconstruction presupposes a fairly sophisticated degree of discrimination and perspicacity, founded on all sorts of experienced . . . distinctions' (Block, 1991: 272). Moreover, in over-emphasising the 'flux' and turning away from or de-emphasising social themes, Block suggests that there is the worrying possibility for social and political life that what would be further enshrined in that life was humankind seen as less makers, creative productive beings engaged in meaningful work, and more beings engaged in mere toil: 'The ideals of *homo faber*, the fabricator of the world, which are permanence, stability, and durability . . . sacrificed to abundance, the ideal of the *animal laborans*' (Arendt, 1958: 126). A similar type of concern also prompts Habermas (1981/1985) to insist on some form of objective grounding being required to save us from unfortunate social and political consequences of the total relativism to which he sees this leading; Norris (1993) expresses similar views when he reveals the 'truth about postmodernity'.

Equally, Schalow (1990) argues against Caputo's rejection of the possibility of answering Heidegger's question of the 'meaning of Being', indicating the misunderstanding of both Heidegger's question and the project he initiates to answer to it. Heidegger had begun *Being and Time* with an analysis of our everyday experience, of the features of life that made up our ordinary understanding of our existence and, implicitly, of 'Being'. 'This exercise of "hermeneutic phenomenology" works from the premise that we all equally possess a "pre-comprehension" or a pre-ontological understanding of being, and that hidden within its deepest folds are the clues for deciphering what is meant by human existence' (Schalow, 1990: 153).

Schalow's observation points us to the practical realm, where the notion of *phronesis* has become important. Gallagher (1993) considers this notion as an important concept for dealing with questions of justice and the moral life in the conditions described by postmodern thinkers; conditions in which epistemology has to deal with paradoxes, inconsistencies, incompleteness, a plurality of narratives and a widespread acceptance of relativism. However postmodern thinking is ultimately evaluated, the concept of *phronesis* is important because through this notion hermeneutics is drawn into the sphere of practical life. *Phronesis* was considered earlier and here it is sufficient to note how the concept is used to give a practical, action-orientation to the understandings derived from the hermeneutic method. As Bubner notes, the practical outcomes always remain unspecificable in detail, but, in general terms, our understanding of the remnants of the past and of the dialogues in which we engage influences us in various ways: 'I may proceed to action, I may alter my life, become a better human being, or merely permit some marginal modifications to my conduct to follow' (1981: 59). Whatever the specifics, the attempt we make is to frame our actions by reference to a 'prudent compromise' between individual needs, wants and interests, and the very real imperatives that we experience as acting on us.

Finally, Redding (1996) has developed insights concerning Hegel and hermeneutics. What Hegel did, he argues, was to follow on from Kant's 'revolution', which had reversed the relation of knower and world in an analogous way as had Copernicus made the sun not the earth the centre of the universe. That is, the knower was made the centre of knowing, rather than the out-there world being the significant source of knowledge; as noted previously, the mind had more to do with it than might first appear. In this move, immediate experience becomes problematic and intersubjective agreement becomes the basis for establishing real knowledge claims. This requires an account of intersubjectivity which Kant had noted, but not developed. Redding argues that what Kant lacked was the approach which hermeneutics can supply, and that this is what Hegel had provided us with. What Hegel had been urging was not the imposition of some complete, fully worked-out system, but the appreciation of the manner in which these newly centred subjects interacted with present and past subjects like themselves. Thus, following Gadamer (1960/1975), he suggests that what Hegel was arguing was that history – understood as something *posited* not *presupposed* – is to be always integrated and reintegrated into the present. At the level of the individual subject,

> in order *for* one to be open to the claims of another's experience, another who is thought of as experiencing the world from within a set of conditions which are partially different from one's own, one must be able to conceive of that other as an intentional subject for whom there is a

world . . . and also *as* an embodied and located 'thing' within the world and subject to its conditions.

(Redding, 1996: 11)

Hegel took the shift that Kant had initiated – that is, primary significance taken away from the 'world' and given to 'mind' – and wedded Kant's insights to hermeneutics as a way of thinking about intentional human subjects.

Whether it was Schleiermacher noting the psychological dimension that has to be accorded weight alongside the grammatical in interpreting texts, or Dilthey highlighting our psychological grounding in a shared form of life, or Heidegger arguing that hermeneutics was the natural mode of being in the world, or Gadamer arguing for degrees of difference among otherwise similarly 'situated' beings, across all of these thinkers, hermeneutics sought to advance our understanding of our subjectivity and its search for understanding through determining the meaning of phenomena.

Now, all of this noted of the development of hermeneutics, the sketch here given is most usefully supplemented by a final development. This is in the work of Frank (1984/1989), previously noted in connection with the problems of the self. Frank states the challenge to which he was responding:

'the spiritual situation' of the age seems to me to demand that we give some thought to a new definition of subjectivity and individuality (which are not one and the same). Both terms denote concepts that are under attack. . . . The fact that time is unfavourably disposed to the subject does not prove anything against its truth.

(1984/1989: 9)

Frank provides a most thoroughgoing attempt to reconcile poststructuralist and hermeneutic positions and identifies three critical areas in which this reconciliation must be achieved. These are the view of history taken by each position, the manner in which subjectivity is dealt with, and the theory of meaning adopted by each.

Frank's argument ranges across a most perceptive reading of such complex thinkers as Derrida, Foucault, Lacan, Deleuze and Lyotard to derive a position which, while it endorses a structural model of meaning, 'insists on the irreducibility of the individual subject, its uniqueness and the singularity of its sense making' (Schwab, 1984/1989: xxxi). In a position analogous to our earlier comments concerning causation being thought of always in terms of 'fields' in which events occur, Frank accepts much of what the structuralists say, but insists, following Schleiermacher, that the meaning of the all-embracing structures identified by structuralism is always given in some concrete context; narrative structure, for example appears as a specific myth told in *this* place in *this* particular way by *this* particular individual. Moreover, in that particular way of telling a different 'sense' emerges from the different styles of the tellers of the narrative in the particular context. Philosophical hermeneutics is addressed to the underlying inherent rationality of human symbol systems as such. A secondary focus is on the manner in which this rationality is actually applied. Here, 'the most important variable is how the individual appropriates the cultural meanings of his or her environmant . . . a reflexive, selective internalization of those meanings' (Schwab, 1984/1989: xxxvii). Whatever the limits on individual interpretation, the individual does appear able to recognise those limits, such recognition being in fact itself part of the hermeneutic activity. Thus, 'reflexivity assumes a limiting function, telling an agent what *not* to try to achieve' (Schwab, 1984/1989: xxxvii).

Personal construct psychology and hermeneutics

There are clear affinities with personal construct psychology in all of the fore-going observations, more especially with those of Frank (1984/1989). Frank's three critical domains of inquiry are quite comfortable ones for personal construct psychology, which is not unhappy with discussion of a longer-range view of humankind, and very centrally concerned with individual meaning-making. As Kelly (1955/1991: I, 4/I, 3) notes, 'the perspective of the centuries rather than the flicker of passing moments' is a more useful focus for under-standing; and what is to be understood is the 'personal way' in which the individual contemplates and gives meaning to his or her life.

Equally, there is a resonance with Frank's positive account of the self previously noted, but also with the theory of meaning Frank sketches in neostructuralism as it reconciles structuralism and hermeneutics. In respect to meaning he draws on Searle's work and notes his view that 'we frequently mean more than we in fact say . . . the meaning of what is said [depending] on something that is not said, namely, *an interpretation* of what is said with a view to a practical, intersubjectively known aim' (Frank, 1984/1989: 392). Interestingly, in terms of earlier observations, Frank also looks to the work of C.S. Peirce as informative for his elaboration of the neostructuralist theory of meaning.

More generally, personal construct psychology, by reason of its unique approach to the study of behaving which focuses on individual meaning, is accessing a fundamental level or dimension of human being. That is, it is not only that this or that individual attempts to make sense of his or her world, but that this sense-making is so entrenched in and characteristic of the general human condition. Understanding is an 'omnipresent phenomenon' lying in 'the everyday', the *Lebenswelt* or 'life-world', the taken-for-granted back-ground which makes possible the proposing of questions and the making of inquiries in the first place (Rosen, 1991: 723).

Hermeneutic philosophy has, then, concerned itself with this matter of understanding and meaning. In Schleiermacher the psychological aspect would sometimes be to the fore, at other times it would assume a background significance. In Dilthey, the dimension of *time* is added, a historical dimen-sion that sees us accessing our own biographies in the context of their significance for understanding contemporary events, as well as accessing the stories and remnants of the lives of others. In such accessing, contemporary others will be most fruitfully engaged if we recognise ourselves in them. Heidegger, amongst other things, also emphasised the dimension of *time*, the manner in which human beings, indeed, life in general, is drawn forward, 'in existing, the human being is governed by what lies ahead' (Bubner, 1981). Underlying all of these matters is the fact that what is common to different understandings of hermeneutics is the centrality of *questioning*. To question is to doubt, to inquire, to interrogate experience and reality, to search for meaning in it (Schalow, 1991: 162).

To be sure, matters are somewhat more complex than the foregoing observations can hope to convey. In respect to every one of the philosophers mentioned there is a veritable avalanche of commentary awaiting anyone who removes one of their books from the shelf. Their special terminologies and technical concepts, their engagement with often unnamed adversaries (frequently Hegel), and the interpenetration of philosophy and linguistics, all make even introductory words addressed to the specific field difficult to construct. Nonetheless, hopefully we have come sufficiently close to the mark of illustrating some of the form or style of hermeneutics sufficient to our purposes.

In the field of personality and clinical psychology, where personal construct psychology has its focus and range of convenience, there is a field where the psychological element is paramount: the 'grammatical' secondary. In that field, there is a view of life characterised by its 'essential measurability in the dimension of time' and the particular value of 'the perspective of the centuries' (Kelly, 1955/1991: I, 8/I, 7; I, 3/I, 3). Moreover, Rowe (1978) reminds us of the essence of personal construct psychology in noting how each of us, in trying to understand our world, structures and evaluates that world, creating a world of meaning. We do this through a system of constructs arising from 'reason, metaphor and myth', meaning-making being a 'fundamental attribute of human beings', with the consequent irony that what we impose meaning on may be in fact 'ultimately and forever meaningless' (Rowe, 1978: 25). Nonetheless, the relentless interrogation of life appears to be our lot.

The affinities between hermeneutics and personal construct psychology, obvious in all of the foregoing observations, are powerful. This may not be surprising given the points of contact between early pragmatism and hermeneutics, and the significance of pragmatism for the development of personal construct psychology.

This said, we should note that what is constructed is not the world, but meaning. For personal construct psychology, the world exists and it exerts an influence on us via the testing of our constructs and the efforts we make to verify them using that very world. We construct meaning in the face of a myriad of unresolved epistemological problems, and while our constructions may be accepted as tentative in terms of their epistemological status, personal construct psychology, *qua* psychology, accepts them as proper objects for investigation, for dialogue. This is perhaps illustrated by our earlier discussion of how Kelly (1955/1991) locates his position within a smaller area of epistemology, characterised as *gnosiology*. His primary focus was on how we *work* with constructs to create meaning, and only secondarily on how this contributes to epistemology proper, and, indeed, how it contributes to the project that is philosophy itself. Yet, 'We have taken the basic view that whatever is characteristic of thought is descriptive of the thinker; that the essentials of scientific curiosity must underlie human curiosity in general' (Kelly, 1955/1991: I, 16/I, 11–12). Thus he goes on to note how philosophy is rooted in the psychological study of human beings, the fundamental, ontological given in all of this being our will to meaning-making.

The contribution of personal construct psychology, as a psychology, to this last level of consideration, this more general feature of our being in the world, invites a final reflection which points us to a final philosophical dimension of personal construct psychology.

Psychological philosophical anthropology

This final dimension is philosophical anthropology, more particularly psychological philosophical anthropology. This is perhaps something of a controversial point in terms of an identification of personal construct psychology with the tradition in which Heidegger is located; Heidegger opposed all forms of philosophical anthropology. Nonetheless, when we get to be talking about meaning in life and of Life, we have moved up a level from that of the individual and find ourselves saying more general things about human beings. This, indeed, did not phase Kelly, who begins his major work with a discussion of man (humanity) not of men or individual man; though the focus on humanity was to illuminate a theory of individual personality.

In its focus on the general dimension of meaning-making, personal construct psychology might be argued to contribute to the broader focus that is psychological philosophical anthropology. We made this suggestion by way of registering a caveat on our caveat, and it is appropriate to return to it here.

Philosophical anthropology links the human sciences in a coordinated fashion to assist the philosophical study of humankind. That study is a critical one, but also synthetic and is focused on Humankind's potentialities; what we could be, rather than what we have been observed to have been or done. Stimulated in conditions of advanced technology which critics had accused of dehumanising human beings and conflating actuality and potentiality, philosophical anthropology has issued in a significant critique of technology. Across different approaches, it invites a critical dialogue with science, sharing the methods of phenomenology and the focus on lived human experience of existentialism.

There are different sub-branches of philosophical anthropology. For example, biological philosophical anthropology examines biological findings and theories in the light of the notion that our cultural achievements are a function of human physiological constitution. Cultural philosophical anthropology places history at the core, scrutinising the record of historical cultural achievement for commonalities. Theological philosophical anthropology addresses the significance of a God who has left options open to a created being. Psychological philosophical anthropology concerns itself with augmenting the findings of experimental psychology with philosophical reflection on the meaning of results therein obtained.

Marcuse, addressing Kant's question 'What is Man?', clarifies the approach of philosophical anthropology:

> The answer to this question is concerned not as the description of human nature as it is actually found to be, but rather as the demonstration of what are found to be human potentialities. In the bourgeois period, philosophy distorted the meaning of both question and answer by equating human potentialities with those that are real within the established order.
>
> (1937/1968: 146)

Pappe (1961) notes in his overview of philosophical anthropology that analyses of particularly human behaviour like laughter, crying, shame, fantasy, fear, resentment, and so forth, have regard not to the stimuli for such behaviour but to the selective and synthesising acts of interpretation that underlie them and give a clue to the essential nature of these behaviours and the understanding they give of our human beingness. In such analyses, phenomenology figures prominently, and what has been a core concern of phenomenology as it developed has been at the heart of personal construct psychology; that is, its concern with *meaning*.

From the perspective of 'psychologic', personal construct psychology provides a thoroughgoing account of the processes of this dimension. Moreover, it well illustrates the difference between logic and psychologic in the modulation corollary. Here, within the *same* construct system there can be construings which are inferentially logically incompatible. The example is of a mother who at one point violently beats her child, at another completely ignores its normal need for attention, at another hugs it, at yet another attends to its basic needs, but over all these behaviours holds on to a construction of herself as a good mother. These apparently contradictory behaviours are held together by this overarching construction in a way that logic would have difficulty with. Psychologic, on the other hand, has little difficulty with this.

Yet, in another way personal construct psychology is more than this. In the simplest form this is given in the manner in which any account of how mind or consciousness functions is illuminated by empirical study of how *this* or *these* minds function. This is how we attempt to derive mata-cognitive theories; we study the activity of the mind in thinking in order to understand what thinking 'is'. Of course, psychology when it gets lost in the empirical loses sight of this, but there is nonetheless value in understanding the actual process of thinking and problem-solving and learning in order to understand their essence.

Now, apart from its affinities with the general existential and humanist traditions which have been most important for psychological philosophical anthropology, personal construct psychology in its original conception drew attention to a number of key themes of philosophical anthropology. The primary significance of the idiographic focus is a most obvious connection to this domain, but there are deeper ones. Kelly suggests that the idiographic approach can be enlarged as a secondary task for the psychologist is to abstract 'from the individual constructs in order to produce constructs which underlie people in general' (1955/1991: I, 43/I, 30). Further, the therapist's urgings for a client to 'articulate his efforts with the enthusiasms of other people so that they may undertake joint enquiries into the nature of life' has the same significance for wider considerations about humanity in general (Kelly, 1955/1991: I, 402/I, 297–8). Most telling, however, is that we not only consider what humankind does, but what it might do, highlighting the focus on *potential* that Marcuse has identified as lying at the core of Kant's question. As Kelly indicates:

> Rather than drawing from their actuarial studies the inference that human initiative is only what it has heretofore been, psychology's greater task is to join mankind in the exploration of what human behavior might be, and what would happen if it were. This is not merely a speculative or an artistic understanding; it can be just as rigorously scientific as the psychology that treats behavior as its dependent variable – indeed, more so.
>
> (1966/1979k: 36)

These observations provide a perception of personal construct psychology that is masked by its primarily idiographic focus. In stressing the meaning-making in which individuals engage there is a focus on the meaning-making activity of human beings generally. Novak (1993) has enlarged and given a detailed account of this last type of general claim. He provides a most significant account of human learning which seeks to unify psychological and epistemological phenomena for a comprehensive understanding of meaning-making. His claim is that all human beings have 'an enormous capacity to make meaning and use language to construct and communicate meanings', and that we can usefully conflate 'issues that deal with the nature of knowledge construction into issues that deal with the psychology of meaning making' (Novak, 1993: 190).

Concluding comment

In making its model of the person that of a scientist, that is, an inquirer, personal construct psychology highlights a feature that has been central in philosophy since Hegel; that is, the manner in which the rediscovered subject comes to understand the world. A sketch of the development of hermeneutics discloses a great deal of similarity between some of the key topics and themes of this important perspective in philosophy and personal construct psychology. An understanding of personal construct psychology as a *hermeneutic constructivism* appears as defensible as an understanding of it as an *epistemological constructivism* (Chiari and Nuzzo, 1996a, 1996b). This takes on added significance when wedded to Butt's (1996) understanding of personal construct psychology as a theory of social action. Hermeneutics, as it has developed and with whatever promise or difficulties, has been taken more and more to the realm of practice and action.

Hermeneutics in philosophy, however, had a deeper reach, particularly in such thinkers as Heidegger. At its deepest level what was to be understood was the nature of Being itself, not merely situations in the world, or situations in which we had our being. Hermeneutics was a philosophical theory of understanding. Hermeneutics in psychology has a more modest focus on the manner in which we seek to understand the world by means of a consciousness which projects itself outwards, that is, expresses intentions. Further, intentional projection is in terms of an ongoing patterning that exerts, and endeavours to maintain, a coherence between new understandings and the existing pattern of meaning. It is also in terms of external reality that we must engage, and engage significantly in its own terms. Thus, if we seek to understand (or help) another, we must do so in terms of our understanding of the wider pattern of meanings through which that other seeks to understand his or her world.

In earlier hermeneutics, this demarcation between the philosophical and the psychological (or sociological) was more marked, and the problem of moving from the *logic of the world*, to the domain of *practice* is only partly overcome through a theory of action (for example, as *phronesis*). Personal construct psychology overcomes this problem by tying understanding to meaning tested in the world of practice and action. As Noaparast (1995) argues, this modifies its hermeneutic harmonies sufficient to allow the identification of personal construct psychology as a realistic constructivism.

It can be assumed with reasonable confidence that Kelly was significantly unaware of developments in European philosophy that led into hermeneutics as it developed. However, while his eminence may have been 'accidental' (Appelbaum, 1969), personal construct psychology is at home with the general orientation of this development. It appears to be particularly at home with recent efforts to negotiate between hermeneutics and poststructuralism (Frank, 1984/1989).

Further, while it is undoubtedly a 'mere' psychology, personal construct psychology has a wider philosophical significance in addressing the domain that is philosophical anthropology. In other words, it is a psychology that is truer to the human condition of situatedness and the growth of knowledge and understanding through our encounters with the meanings that others construct.

Conclusion

Personal construct psychology, since its original formulation by Kelly in the first half of this century, appears to have weathered well the storms that have buffeted philosophy and psychology from that time. It is, as we have seen, a psychology and not a philosophy, and it cannot be expected to provide answers to the traditional problems with which this latter discipline has been centrally concerned. Nevertheless, it sits well with a philosophical tradition of some considerable integrity which continues to be reaccessed in contemporary philosophy, as well as in the human sciences, for the insights it provides. The original location of personal construct psychology in terms of 'the types of philosophical systems with which scholars are familiar' (Kelly 1955/1991: I, 16/I, 12) did not lock it in preemptively to a too narrow perspective and it has proven to have accessed ideas that have been most durable and highly pertinent to advanced thinking in contemporary social and psychological theory. This is even more so in respect of the less explicit, 'latent' philosophical dimensions of personal construct psychology.

Within a plethora of constructionisms and constructivisms, personal construct psychology appears to generate most anxiety for the social constructionists. Significant in this is the matter of the *self*. However, a review of thinking about this notion suggests that the general consensus of self as *process*, or more sophisticatedly as a *self-organising* systemic process, is quite compatible with personal construct psychology. Further, an elaboration of the sociality and commonality corollaries in the direction of greater account being taken of the social realm (whatever that turns out to be) and the role of language (whatever best account of language emerges from the efforts of the linguists and the philosophers of language) appears well accommodated by personal construct psychology. This can be argued specifically in terms of its content, and in terms of its own humility as a theory; that is, its invitation to use it, modify it, and move on. This appears less true of social constructionism, which is in some respects but a more sophisticated form of the type of social theory that Marx had advanced, and which may be open to the same criticisms that are well rehearsed in decades of scholarship in philosophy; notwithstanding Marx's most illuminating insights concerning social life generally. In the event, social constructionism is less conciliatory toward personal construct psychology than the latter is to the concerns of the social constructionists. As we have noted, personal construct psychology is the only theory of psychology *and* psychotherapy (Chiari and Nuzzo, 1996a), the only psychology for psychotherapy which also was based on human interaction (Mair, 1970a), and might be in fact best thought of as a theory of 'social action' (Butt, 1996).

The phenomenon that is postmodernism has touched most areas of human life and thought and it appears to have profound implications for psychology. However, when these implications are considered 'up close', they appear less radical than they do at first sight, and a practical response by psychology seems less urgent. Whatever the final outcome of a mapping of the diverse 'charts' produced by postmodernity onto the territory of psychology in general, personal construct psychology appears better placed than most perspectives to emerge without too much of its territory ceded. It does appear to avoid and evade most of the criticisms of psychology made from within postmodernism, with a notable exception; that is, its stress on the individual. This alleged overstress on the individual weakens as a criticism, however, with a fuller understanding of personal construct psychology as significantly an interpersonal psychology. Equally, it might be seen to weaken in the absence of an adequate psychology for postmodernism. This is not to say that such a psychology will not emerge; Shotter (1997), for example, has made a particularly strong claim for a psychology developing out of social constructionism. However, it would appear at this stage that the best we can do is to revert to the analogy of two different searchlights illuminating the same territory of human behaving, the fruits of the understandings thus obtained taken in accord with a principle of 'complementarity' (Rychlak, 1993).

Advanced thinking in cognitive science (particularly the renewed importance of 'the subjective'), in philosophy of science for psychology (for example, the continued insistence on a humanistic approach), in psychology itself when it recognises the demise of a real psychology of personality (for example, the loss of the 'person' in psychology of personality), and in psychotherapy (replacing 'adjustment' with 'change') all find a congenial fit with personal construct psychology. Moreover, personal construct psychology, while it might make itself relatively politically impotent thereby and also open to a charge of being ideological, assumes an open, non-exploitative social-political context which in its own practice it contributes toward. It offers also a way of understanding spiritual belief that is in this same egalitarian mode, perhaps highlighting an outlook that was closer to the ethic of love that Hegel finds to be the true message of Jesus and which he characterises as the *ethical life*. This is the opposite to religion as dogma, a position that others have observed was true also of Kelly's own religious beliefs (Fransella, 1995: 22) and has positive rather than negative social-political implications.

Finally, there is not only a contribution to our thinking about the functioning of the individual as such, and about individuals functioning together in community and society, but also to the questions of human potential; that is, to the bigger questions of the nature of human beings and our place in the world. Personal construct psychology, by commencing with a location of itself within traditional philosophical systems, and, more so, by grounding itself in a systematic philosophical position, that is, constructive alternativism, moves this psychology into a larger domain, that of philosophical anthropology. If psychology is able to pause from its obsession with data collection and refocus on the task of formulating concepts that might genuinely advance our understanding of human beings, it will find personal construct psychology a most friendly ally and a forerunner of such a project.

If this sounds all a bit to good to be true, then so be it. There is always a danger of inflating a particular and limited theory into a 'religio-philosophical system', as Kelly (1955/1991: I, 11/I, 8) observed of Freud's work. Indeed, in such an inflation, inconsistencies are likely to be noted as 'what is reasonably true within one limited range is not quite so true outside that range' (1955/1991: I, 11/I, 8).

Thus with the present volume. We have attempted to engage with the wide range of more abstract and ultimate matters that philosophy has concerned itself with. The fact that such an engagement can be so productively made confirms the range of matters in respect of which one might take a 'personal construct psychology viewpoint'. This does not imply that the range of the miniature system that is personal construct psychology has been enlarged. Rather, the suggestion is more modest. It is, simply, that those who find in personal construct psychology a valuable approach to their own understanding of understanding – their own, and others', and their own 'of' others – can take an added degree of comfort in the fact that it appears well aligned with a substantial philosophical tradition, and has something interesting to say to a range of matters of interest to philosophers, and/or is open to interesting things that philosophers say to psychologists.

While there is no intention to inflate personal construct psychology into a 'religio-philosophical system', the inconsistencies that Kelly warns of when this is done may well have appeared in this volume nonetheless. That being so, it is well to reiterate that this work itself represents a personal construction and a conversation with personal construct psychology in the field of issues that have been of common concern to philosophers and personal construct psychologists. Realism and constructivism may be odd bedfellows, some approaches within phenomenology may be totally opposed to any form of anthropology, the self (or selves) as understood by postmodern thought may be less rather than more compatible with the self in personal construct psychology, and so on. Nonetheless, an articulation of personal construct psychology in terms of the themes and issues here discussed is coherent within at least one personal construct system, and hopefully provocative of both validation and invalidation in those of others.

References

Ackermann, R. (1965) *Theories of Knowledge: A Critical Introduction*, New York: McGraw-Hill Inc.

Adams-Webber, J. (1990) 'Personal Construct Theory and Cognitive Science', *International Journal of Personal Construct Psychology*, 3: 415–21.

Adams-Webber, J. and Mancuso, J.C. (eds) (1983) *Applications of Personal Construct Theory*, London: Academic Press.

Adorno, T.W., Frenkel-Brunswick, E., Levison, D.F. and Sanford, R.N. (1950) *The Authoritarian Personality*, New York: Harper and Row.

Althusser, L. (1971) *Lenin and Philosophy and Other Essays*, New York: New Left Books.

Anderson, J. (1960) 'Critical Notice: Time and Idea: The Theory of History of Giambattista Vico', *Australian Journal of Philosophy*, 38: 166–72.

—— (1962) *Studies in Empirical Philosophy*, Sydney: Angus and Robertson.

Appelbaum, S.A. (1969) 'The Accidental Eminence of George Kelly', *Psychiatry and Social Science Review*, 3: 20–5.

Arendt, H. (1958) *The Human Condition*, Chicago: University of Chicago Press.

Armstrong, D. (1968) *A Materialist Theory of Mind*, London: Routledge and Kegan Paul.

—— (1977) 'On Metaphysics', *Quadrant*, July: 65–9.

Baker, A.J. (1979) *Anderson's Social Philosophy*, Sydney: Angus and Robertson.

—— (1986) *Australian Realism: The Systematic Philosophy of John Anderson*, London: Cambridge University Press.

Balbi, J. (1996) 'What is a Person? Reflections on the Domain of Psychology from an Ontological and Postrationalist Perspective', *Journal of Constructivist Psychology*, 9: 249–62.

Baldwin, J.M. (ed.) (1960) *Dictionary of Psychology and Philosophy*, Gloucester, Mass.: Peter Smith. Original work published 1906.

Bannister, D. (1970) 'Psychological Theories as Ways of Relating to People', *British Journal of Medical Psychology*, 43(3): 241–4.

—— (1983) 'Self in Personal Construct Theory', in J. Adams-Webber and J.C. Mancuso (eds), *Applications of Personal Construct Theory*, Toronto: Academic Press.

Bannister, D. and Fransella, F. (1971) *Inquiring Man*, Harmondsworth: Penguin.

Bannister, D., Fransella, F. and Agnew, J. (1971) 'Characteristics and Validity of the GRID TEST of Thought Disorder', *British Journal of Clinical Psychology*, 10: 144–51.

Bannister, D. and Mair, J.M.M. (1968) *The Evaluation of Personal Constructs*, London: Academic Press.

Barbu, Z. (1956) *Democracy and Dictatorship: Their Psychology and Patterns of Life*, London: Routledge.

—— (1960) *Problems of Historical Psychology*, London: Routledge.

—— (1971) *Society, Culture and Personality*, New York: Schocken Books.

Barclay, C.R. and Smith, T.S. (1993) 'Autobiographical Remembering and Self-Composing', *International Journal of Personal Construct Psychology*, 6: 1–26.

Barglow, R. (1994) *The Crisis of the Self in the Age of Information*, London: Routledge.

Barth, K. (1982) *The Theology of Schleiermacher*, translated by G.W. Bromley, edited by D. Ritschl, Edinburgh: T. and T. Clark. Original lectures delivered 1923–4.

Barthes, R. (1967) *Elements of Semiology*, translated by A. Lavers and C. Smith, London: Jonathan Cape. Original work published 1964 in French.

—— (1973) *Mythologies*, translated by A. Lavers, London: Jonathan Cape. Original work published 1957 in French.

Baum, R.F. (1988) *Doctors of Modernity: Darwin, Marx and Freud*, Peru, Ill.: Sherwood Sugden and Company.

de Beauvoir, S. (1975) 'Interview with Pierre Vicary', in M. Charlesworth, *The Existentialists and Jean-Paul Sartre*, Brisbane: University of Queensland Press.

Berger, P.L. and Luckmann, T. (1966), *The Social Construction of Reality*, New York: Doubleday Inc.

Bernstein, R.J. (1972) *Praxis and Action*, London: Duckworth.

—— (1983) *Beyond Objectivism and Relativism: Science, Hermeneutics, and Practice*, Oxford: Blackwell.

Berzonsky, M.D. (1989) 'The Self as a Theorist: Individual Differences in Identity Formation', *International Journal of Personal Construct Psychology*, 2: 363–76.

—— (1990) 'Self-construction over the Lifespan: A Process Perspective on Identity Formation', in G.J. Neimeyer and R.A. Neimeyer (eds), *Advances in Personal Construct Theory, Vol. 1*, Greenwich, Conn.: JAI Press.

Bickhard, M.H. (1993) 'On why Constructivism Does Not Yield Relativism', *Journal of Theoretical Artificial Intelligence*, 5: 275–84.

—— (1996) 'Troubles with Computationalism', in W. O'Donohue and R.F. Kitchener (eds), *The Philosophy of Psychology*, London: Sage.

Block, E. (Jr) (1991) 'Radical Hermeneutics as Radical Homelessness', *Philosophy Today*, 35: 269–76.

Block, N. (ed.) (1980) *Readings in Philosophy of Psychology*, London: Methuen (two volumes).

Bolton, N. (1979) 'Phenomenology and Education', *British Journal of Educational Studies*, 27: 245–58.

Botella, L. (1995) 'Personal Construct Psychology, Constructivism, and Postmodern Thought', in R.A. Neimeyer and G.J. Neimeyer (eds), *Advances in Personal Construct Psychology, Vol. 3*, New York: JAI Press.

Brenkert, G. (1983) *Marx's Ethics of Freedom*, London: Routledge.

Bridgman, P.W. (1927) *The Logic of Modern Physics*, New York: Macmillan.

Broad, C.D. (1962) *Five Types of Ethical Theory*, London: Routledge and Kegan Paul. Original work published 1930.

Brown, P. (1973) *Radical Psychology*, London: Tavistock Publications.

Brown, S.C. (1974) *Philosophy of Psychology*, London: The Macmillan Press Ltd.

Bubner, R. (1981) *Modern German Philosophy*, Cambridge: Cambridge University Press.

Bugental, J.F.T. (1980) 'Being Levels of Therapeutic Growth', in R.N. Walsh and F. Vaughan (eds), *Beyond Ego*, Los Angeles: J.P. Tarcher.

Bugental, J.F.T. and Bugental, E.K. (1984) 'A Fate Worse than Death: The Fear of Changing', *Psychotherapy*, 21: 543–9.

Bunge, M. (1976) 'The Philosophical Richness of Technology', in *Proceedings of the Philosophy of Science Association*, 2: 185–93.

Bunge, M. and Ardila, R. (1987) *Philosophy of Psychology*, New York: Springer-Verlag.

Burkitt, I. (1996) 'Social and Personal Constructs: A Division Left Unresolved', *Theory and Psychology*, 6(1): 71–7.

Burnett, J. (1968) *Greek Philosophy: Thales to Plato*, London: Macmillan. Original work published 1914.

Butt, T. (1996), 'PCP: Cognitive or Social Psychology', in J.W. Scheer and A. Catina (eds), *Empirical Constructivism in Europe: The Personal Construct Approach*, Giessen: Psychosozial-Verlag.

—— (1997) 'The Existentialism of George Kelly', *Journal of the Society for Existential Analysis*, 8: 20–32.

—— (1998a) 'Sedimentation and Elaborative Choice', *Journal of Constructivist Psychology*. In press.

—— (1998b) 'Sociality and Embodiment', *Journal of Constructivist Psychology*. In press.

Button, E. (ed.) (1985) *Personal Construct Theory and Mental Health*, London: Croom Helm.

Campbell, N.R. (1957) *Foundations of Science: The Philosophy of Theory and Experiment*, New York: Dover.

Caputo, J.D. (1987) *Radical Hermeneutics*, Bloomington: University of Indiana Press.

Carroll, J. (1974) *Breakout from the Crystal Palace*, London: Routledge and Kegan Paul.

Chaiklin, S. (1992) 'From Theory to Practice and Back Again: What Does Postmodern Philosophy Contribute to Psychological Science?', in S. Kvale (ed.), *Psychology and Postmodernism*, London: Sage Publications.

Chalmers, D.J. (1996) 'Facing up to the Problem of Consciousness', in S.R. Hameroff, A.W. Kaszniak and A.C. Scott (eds), *Toward a Science of Consciousness*, Cambridge, Mass.: MIT Press.

Charlesworth, M. (1975) *The Existentialists and Jean-Paul Sartre*, Brisbane: University of Queensland Press.

Chiari, G. and Nuzzo, M.L. (1996a) 'Personal Construct Theory Within Psychological Constructivism: Precursor or Avant-Garde?', in B.M. Walker, J. Costigan, L.L. Viney and B. Warren (eds), *Personal Construct Theory: A Psychology for the Future*, Melbourne: Australian Psychological Society.

—— (1996b) 'Psychological Constructivisms: A Metatheoretical Differentiation', *Journal of Constructivist Psychology*, 9: 163–86.

Cohen, A. and Dascal, M. (1991) *The Institution of Philosophy: A Discipline in Crisis?*, La Salle, Ill.: Open Court Publishing Company. Original work published 1989.

Colapietro, V.M. (1990) 'The Vanishing Subject of Contemporary Discourse', *The Journal of Philosophy*, LXXXVII: 644–55.

Comte, A. (1908) *A General View of Positivism*, translated by J.H. Bridges with an introduction by F. Harrison, London: George Routledge and Sons. Original work published 1848 in French.

Corsini, R.J. (ed.) (1994) *Encyclopedia of Psychology*, New York: John Wiley and Sons.

Cox, L.M. and Lyddon, W.J. (1997) 'Constructivist Conceptions of Self: A Discussion of Emerging Identity Constructs', *Journal of Constructivist Psychology*, 10: 201–20.

Crites, S. (1971) 'The Narrative Quality of Experience', *Journal of the American Academy of Religion*, 39: 293–311.

Cushman, P. (1990) 'Why the Self is Empty: Toward a Historically Situated Psychology', *American Psychologist*, 45: 599–611.

Dalton, P. and Dunnett, G. (1990) *A Psychology for Living: Personal Construct Theory for Professional Practice*, London: Dunton Publishing.

Davies, P. (1992) *The Mind of God*, London: Simon and Schuster.

Derrida, J. (1973) *Speech and Phenomena and Other Essays on Husserl's Theory of Signs*, translated by D.B. Allison, Evanston, Ill.: Northwestern University Press. Original work published 1967 in French.

—— (1976) *Of Grammatology*, translated by G.C. Spivak, Baltimore: Johns Hopkins University Press. Original work published 1967 in French.

Deutscher, M. (1983) *Subjecting and Objecting*, Brisbane: University of Queensland Press.

Dewey, J. (1966) *Democracy and Education*, New York: Free Press. Original work published 1916.

—— (1968) 'The Development of American Pragmatism', in his *Philosophy and Civilization*, Gloucester, Mass.: Peter Smith. Original work published 1932.

Dilthey, W. (1976) *Selected Writings*, translated and edited by H.P. Rickman, Cambridge: Cambridge University Press.

Doniela, B. (1984) 'The Frankfurt School's Notion of Rationality', *Dialectic* (University of Newcastle, Australia), 23: 84–92.

Duck, S. (1983) 'Sociality and Cognition in Personal Construct Theory', in J. Adams-Webber and J. Mancuso (eds), *Applications of Personal Construct Theory*, Toronto: Academic Press.

Durbin, P.T. (1976) 'Are There Interesting Philosophical Issues in Technology as Distinct from Science?', *Proceedings of the Philosophy of Science Association*, 2: 139–71.

D'Urso, S. (1971) *Counterpoints: Critical Writing on Australian Education*, Sydney: J. Wiley and Sons, Australia.

Edwards, P. (ed.) (1972) *The Encyclopedia of Philosophy*, New York: Macmillan Publishing Company.

Ellul, J. (1965) *The Technological Society*, translated by J. Wilkinson, London: Jonathan Cape. Original work published 1954 in French.

—— (1980) *The Technological System*, translated by J. Neugroschel, New York: The Continuum Publishing Corporation. Original work published 1977 in French.

Epting, F.R., and Amerikaner, M. (1980) 'Optimal Functioning : A Personal Construct Approach', in A.W. Landfield and L.M. Leitner (eds), *Personal Construct Psychology: Psychotherapy and Personality*, New York: Wiley International.

Epting, F.R., Prichard, S., Leitner, L.M. and Dunnett, G. (1996) 'Personal Constructions of the Social', in D. Kalekin-Fishman and B.M. Walker (eds), *The
Construction of Group Realities*, Malabar, Fla: Krieger Publishing Company.

Erwin, E. (1978) *Behaviour Therapy: Scientific, Philosophical and Moral Foundations*,
Cambridge: Cambridge University Press.

Feyerabend, P. (1975) *Against Method*, London: New Left Books.

Flanagan, O. (1996) 'Deconstructing Dreams: The Spandrels of Sleep', in S.R.
Hameroff, A.W. Kaszniak and A.C. Scott (eds), *Toward a Science of Consciousness*,
Cambridge, Mass.: MIT Press.

Floistad, G. (ed.) (1981) *Contemporary Philosophy, Vol. 1*, The Hague: Martinus
Nijhoff Publishers.

Flugel, J.C. (1955) *Man, Morals and Society*, Harmondsworth: Penguin.

Ford, K.M., Hayes, P.J. and Adams-Webber, J. (1993) 'The Missing Link: A Reply to
Joseph Rychlak', *International Journal of Personal Construct Psychology*, 6: 313–26.

Foster, H. (ed.) (1985) *Postmodern Culture*, London: Pluto Press.

Foucault, M. (1977) *Madness and Civilization*, translated by R. Howard, London:
Tavistock Publications. Original work published 1961 in French.

—— (1982) 'The Subject and Power', *Critical Inquiry*, 8: 777–95.

—— (1988) 'The Dangerous Individual', in L.D. Kritzman (ed.), *Michel Foucault:
Politics, Philosophy, Culture: Interviews and Other Writings 1977–1984*, London:
Routledge. Original essay published 1978 in French.

—— (1993) 'About the Beginnings of the Hermeneutics of the Self', *Political Theory*,
21: 198–227.

Frank, M. (1989) *What is Neostructuralism?*, translated by S. Wilke and R. Gray,
Minneapolis: University of Minnesota Press. Original work published 1984 in
German.

Frankena, W. (1970) 'A Model for Analyzing a Philosophy of Education', in J.R.
Martin (ed.), *Readings in the Philosophy of Education*, Boston: Allyn and Bacon
Inc.

Frankl, V.E. (1962) *Man's Search for Meaning*, New York: Simon and Schuster.

—— (1967) *Psychotherapy and Existentialism*, Harmondsworth: Penguin.

Fransella, F. (1983) 'What Sort of Person is the Person as Scientist', in J. Adams-
Webber and J.C. Mancuso (eds), *Applications of Personal Construct Theory*,
London: Academic Press.

—— (1995) *George Kelly*, London: Sage Publications.

Freire, P. (1972a) *Cultural Action for Freedom*, Harmondsworth: Penguin.

—— (1972b) *Pedagogy of the Oppressed*, Harmondsworth: Penguin.

Friedman, M. (1995) 'Constructivism, Psychotherapy, and the Dialogue of Touchstones', *Journal of Constructivist Psychology*, 8: 283–92.

Fromm, E. (1942) *The Fear of Freedom*, London: Routledge.

—— (1968) *The Sane Society*, London: Routledge. Original work published 1956.

Gadamer, H.G. (1975) *Truth and Method*, London: Sheed and Ward. Original work
published 1960.

Galin, D. (1996) 'The Structure of Subjective Experience: Sharpen the Concepts and
Terminology', in S.R. Hameroff, A.W. Kaszniak and A.C. Scott (eds), *Toward a
Science of Consciousness*, Cambridge, Mass.: MIT Press.

Gallagher, S. (1993) 'The Place of Phronesis in Postmodern Hermeneutics', *Philosophy
Today*, 37: 298–305.

Gallie, W.B. (1952) *Peirce and Pragmatism*, Harmondsworth: Penguin.

Gardner, H. (1985) *The Mind's New Science: A History of the Cognitive Revolution*, New York: Basic Books.

Gergen, K.J. (1985) 'The Social Constructionist Movement in Modern Psychology', *American Psychologist*, 40: 266–75.

—— (1989a) 'Social Psychology and the Wrong Revolution', *European Journal of Social Psychology*, 19: 463–84.

—— (1989b) 'Warranting Voices and the Elaboration of the Self', in J. Shotter and K.J. Gergen (eds), *Texts of Identity*, Newbury Park, Calif.: Sage Publications.

—— (1991) *The Saturated Self*, New York: Basic Books.

—— (1992) 'Toward a Postmodern Psychology', in S. Kvale (ed.), *Psychology and Postmodernism*, London: Sage Publications.

—— (1994) 'Emotion as Relationship', in K.J. Gergen (ed.), *Realities and Relationships*, Cambridge, Mass.: Harvard University Press.

—— (1997) 'On the Poly/tics of Postmodern Psychology', *Theory & Psychology*, 7: 31–6.

Giorgi, A. (1981) 'On the Relationship Among the Psychologist's Fallacy, Psychologism, and the Phenomenological Reduction', *Journal of Phenomenological Psychology*, 12: 75–86.

Glasersfeld, E. von (1995) *Radical Constructivism*, London: Falmer Press.

Gonçalves, O.F. (1995), 'Hermeneutics, Constructivism, and Cognitive-Behavioural Therapies: From the Object to the Project', in R.A. Neimeyer and M.J. Mahoney (eds), *Constructivism and Psychotherapy*, Washington, DC: American Psychological Association.

Gramsci, A. (1975) *Letters From Prison*, London: Jonathan Cape. Original work published 1965 in Italian.

Greene, M. (1970) 'Foreword', in H. Plessner, *Laughing and Crying: A Study of the Limits of Human Behaviour*, translated by J.P. Churchill and M. Greene, Evanston, Ill.: University of Illinois Press.

Habermas, J. (1971) *Knowledge and Human Interests*, translated by J.J. Shapiro, Boston: Beacon Press.

—— (1984) *The Theory of Communicative Action, Vol. 1: Reason and the Rationalization of Society*, translated by T. McCarthy, Boston: Beacon Press. Original work published 1981 in German.

—— (1985) 'Modernity – an Incomplete Project', in H. Foster (ed.), *Postmodern Culture*, London: Pluto Press. Original work published 1981.

—— (1987) *The Theory of Communicative Action, Vol. 2: Lifeworld and System: A Critique of Functional Reason*, translated by T. McCarthy, Boston: Beacon Press. Original work published 1981 in German.

Hameroff, S.R., Kaszniak, A.W. and Scott, A.C. (eds) (1996) *Toward a Science of Consciousness*, Cambridge, Mass.: MIT Press.

Hampshire, S. (1951) *Spinoza*, Harmondsworth: Pelican.

Hardison, O.B. (Jr) (1972) *Towards Freedom and Dignity*, Baltimore: Johns Hopkins University Press.

Harré, R. and Gillett, G. (1994) *The Discursive Mind*, Thousand Oaks, Calif.: Sage Publications.

Harriman, P.L. (1946) *Encyclopedia of Psychology*, New York: Citadel Press.

Harris, K. (1979) *Education and Knowledge: The Structured Misrepresentation of Reality*, London: Routledge and Kegan Paul.

Harris, R. (1996) *The Language Connection*, Bristol: Thoemmes Press.

Hawking, S.W. (1988) *A Brief History of Time*, London: Bantam Books.

Hegel, F. (1961) *On Christianity: Early Theological Writings*, New York: Harper. Original work published 1798–9 in German.

Heidegger, M. (1968) *What is Called Thinking?*, translated by F.D. Wieck and J.G. Gray, New York: Harper and Row. Original work published 1954 in German.

—— (1977) *The Question Concerning Technology*, translated with an introduction by W. Lovitt, New York: Harper and Row. Original work published 1954 in German.

—— (1978) *Being and Time*, translated by J. Macquarrie and E. Robinson, Oxford: Basil Blackwell. Original work published 1927 in German.

Held, B.S. (1995) 'The Real Meaning of Constructivism', *Journal of Constructivist Psychology*, 8: 305–16.

Henle, M. (1986) 'Kurt Lewin as Meta-Theorist', in M. Henle (ed.), *1879 and All That: Essays in the Theory and History of Psychology*, New York: Columbia University Press.

Herbart, J. (1891) *Textbook in Psychology*, translated by M.K. Smith. Original work published 1834 in German.

—— (1977) *The Science of Education*, translated by H.M. Felkin and E. Felkin, edited by D.N. Robinson, Washington, DC: University Publications of America. Original work published 1806 in German.

Hillner, K.P. (1987) *Psychology's Compositional Problem*, Amsterdam: Elsevier Science Publishers.

Holland, R. (1970) 'George Kelly: Constructive Innocent and Reluctant Existentialist', in D. Bannister (ed.), *Perspectives in Personal Construct Theory*, London: Academic Press.

—— (1981) 'From Perspectives to Reflexivity', in H. Bonarius, R. Holland and S. Rosenberg (eds), *Personal Construct Psychology: Recent Advances in Theory and Practice*, Basingstoke: Macmillan.

Hooker, C.A. (1995) *Reason, Regulation and Realism*, Albany, NY: State University of New York Press.

—— (1996) 'Toward a Naturalized Cognitive Science: A Framework for Cooperation Between Philosophy and the Natural Sciences of Intelligent Systems', in W. O'Donohue and R.F. Kitchener (eds), *The Philosophy of Psychology*, London: Sage Publications.

Howard, G.S. (1986) *Dare We Develop a Human Science?* Notre Dame, Ind.: Academic Publications.

—— (1991) *Culture Tales: A Narrative Approach to Thinking, Cross-cultural Psychology, and Psychotherapy*, New York: Guilford Press.

—— (1997) 'Constructive Realism', paper presented to the Twelfth International Conference on Personal Construct Psychology, Seattle.

Howard, G.S., Myers, P.R. and Curtin, T.D. (1991) 'Can Science Furnish Evidence of Human Freedom? Self-determination Versus Conformity in Human Action', *International Journal of Personal Construct Psychology*, 4: 371–95.

Huang, Y. (1996) 'The Father of Hermeneutics in a Postmodern Age', *Philosophy Today*, 40: 251–62.

Hundert, E.M. (1995) *Lessons from an Optical Illusion: On Nature and Nurture, Knowledge and Values*, Cambridge, Mass.: Harvard University Press.

Husain, M. (1983) 'To What Can One Apply A Construct?' In J. Adams-Webber and J.C. Mancuso (eds), *Applications of Personal Construct Theory*, London: Academic Press.

Husserl, E. (1965) *Philosophy and the Crisis of European Man*, translated with an introduction by Q. Lauer, New York: Harper and Row. Original work published 1954 in German.

Jahoda, M. (1988) 'The Range of Convenience of Personal Construct Psychology: An Outsider's View', in F. Fransella and L. Thomas (eds), *Experimenting With Personal Construct Psychology*, London: Routledge.

James, W. (1907a) *A Textbook of Psychology*, London: Macmillan and Co. Limited.

—— (1907b) *Talks to Teachers on Psychology: And to Students on Some of Life's Ideals*, London: Longmans, Green, and Co.

—— (1978) *Pragmatism*, Cambridge, Mass.: Harvard University Press. Original work published 1907.

Jennings, J.L. (1986) 'Husserl Revisited: The Forgotten Distinction Between Psychology and Phenomenology', *American Psychologist*, 41: 1231–40.

John, I.D. and Soyland, A.J. (1990) 'What is the Epistemic Status of the Theory of Personal Constructs?', *International Journal of Personal Construct Psychology*, 3: 51–62.

Johnson, G.A. (1993) 'Ontology and Painting: "Eye and Mind"', in G.A. Johnson (ed.), *The Merleau-Ponty Aesthetics Reader: Philosophy and Painting*, Evanston, Ill.: Northwestern University Press.

Jones, H.G. (1971) 'In Search of an Idiographic Psychology', *Bulletin of the British Psychological Society*, 24: 279–90.

Jung, C.G. (1953) 'Individuation', in *Collected Works, Vol. 7*, translated by R.F.C. Hull, edited by H. Read, M. Fordham and G. Adler, London: Routledge. Original essay published 1945 in German.

Jung, M. (1995) 'From Dilthey to Mead and Heidegger: Systematic and Historical Relations', *Journal of the History of Philosophy*, 33(4): 661–77.

Kalekin-Fishman, D. (1995) 'Kelly and Issues of Power', *Journal of Constructivist Psychology*, 8(1): 19–32.

Kalekin-Fishman, D. and Walker, B.M. (1996) *The Construction of Group Realities*, Malabar, Fla: Krieger Publishing Company.

Kamenka, E. (1965) 'Marxism and the History of Philosophy', *History and Theory*, 5: 83–104.

Kant, I. (1964) *Critique of Pure Reason*, translated by N.K. Smith, London: Macmillan and Co. Ltd. Original second edition work published 1787 in German.

Kelly, G.A. (1963) *A Theory of Personality: The Psychology of Personal Constructs*, New York: W.W. Norton and Co.

—— (1970) 'A Brief Introduction to Personal Construct Psychology', in D. Bannister (ed.), *Perspectives in Personal Constructs Theory*, London: Academic Press.

—— (1979a) 'Man's Construction of His Alternatives', in B. Maher (ed.), *Clinical Psychology and Personality*, Huntington, NY: Robert E. Krieger Publishing Company. Original essay published 1958.

—— (1979b) 'Personal Construct Theory and the Psychotherapeutic Interview', in B. Maher (ed.), *Clinical Psychology and Personality*, Huntington, NY: Robert E. Krieger Publishing Company. Original essay published 1958.

—— (1979c) 'A Mathematical Approach to Psychology', in B. Maher (ed.) *Clinical Psychology and Personality*, Huntington, NY: Robert E. Krieger Publishing Company. Original essay published 1961.

—— (1979d) 'Sin and Psychotherapy', in B. Maher (ed.), *Clinical Psychology and Personality*, Huntington, NY: Robert E. Krieger Publishing Company. Original essay published 1962.

—— (1979e) 'In Whom Confide: On Whom Depend for What?', in B. Maher (ed.), *Clinical Psychology and Personality*, Huntingdon, NY: Robert E. Krieger Publishing Company. Original essay published 1962.

—— (1979f) 'The Autobiography of a Theory', in B. Maher (ed.), *Clinical Psychology and Personality*, Huntingdon, NY: Robert E. Krieger Publishing Company. Original essay published 1963.

—— (1979g) 'Psychotherapy and the Nature of Man', in B. Maher (ed.), *Clinical Psychology and Personality*, Huntingdon, NY: Robert E. Krieger Publishing Company. Original essay published 1958.

—— (1979h) 'The Language of Hypothesis: Man's Psychological Instrument', in B. Maher (ed.), *Clinical Psychology and Personality*, Huntington, NY: Robert E. Krieger Publishing Company. Original essay published 1964.

—— (1979i) 'The Psychotherapeutic Relationship', in B. Maher (ed.), *Clinical Psychology and Personality*, Huntington, NY: Robert E. Krieger Publishing Company. Original essay published 1965.

—— (1979j) 'The Role of Classification in Personality Theory', in B. Maher (ed.), *Clinical Psychology and Personality*, Huntington, NY: Robert E. Krieger Publishing Company. Original essay published 1965.

—— (1979k) 'Ontological Acceleration', in B. Maher (ed.), *Clinical Psychology and Personality*, Huntington, NY: Robert E. Krieger Publishing Company. Original essay published 1966.

—— (1979l) 'Humanistic Methodology in Psychological Research', in B. Maher (ed.), *Clinical Psychology and Personality*, Huntington, NY: Robert E. Krieger Publishing Company. Original essay published 1966.

—— (1991) *The Psychology of Personal Constructs*, London: Routledge. Original work published New York: W.W. Norton and Co., 1955. (Both editions in two volumes.)

—— (1996) 'Europe's Matrix of Decision', in D. Kalekin-Fishman and B.M. Walker (eds), *The Construction of Group Realities*, Malabar, Fla: Robert E. Krieger Publishing Company. Original essay published 1962.

Kendall, G. and Michael, M. (1997) 'Politicizing the Politics of Postmodern Social Psychology', *Theory & Psychology*, 7: 7–30.

Kendler, H.I. (1981) *Psychology: A Science in Conflict*, New York: Oxford University Press.

Kierkegaard, S. (1980) 'The Sickness Unto Death', in *Kierkegaard's Writings, Vol. XIX*, Princeton: Princeton University Press. Original essay published 1849 in Danish.

Koch, S. (1973) 'The Image of Man in Encounter Groups', *The American Scholar*, 42: 636–52.

Kodis, J. (1896) 'Some Remarks Upon Apperception', *Psychological Review*, 3(4): 384–97.

Kolakowski, L. (1969) *Marxism and Beyond: On Historical Understanding and Individual Responsibility*, translated by J.Z. Peel, London: Granada. Original work published 1957 in Polish.

—— (1971) *Main Currents of Marxism*, translated by P.S. Falla, Oxford: Clarendon Press.

Krippendorf, K. (1991) 'Reconstructing (Some) Communication Research Methods', in F. Steier (ed.), *Research and Reflexivity*, London: Sage Publications.

Krishna, D. (1965) *Considerations Towards a Theory of Social Change*, Bombay: Manaktalas and Sons.

Kropotkin, P. (1902) *Mutual Aid*, London: Heinemann.

Kuhn, T. (1970) *The Structure of Scientific Revolutions*, second revised edition, Chicago: University of Chicago Press. Original work published 1962.

Kvale, S. (1992) *Psychology and Postmodernism*, London: Sage Publications.

Lakatos, I. (1970) 'Falsification and Methodology in Social Science', in I. Lakatos and A. Musgrave (eds), *Criticism and the Growth of Knowledge*, Cambridge: Cambridge University Press.

Lakatos, I. and Musgrave, A. (eds) (1970) *Criticism and the Growth of Knowledge*, Cambridge: Cambridge University Press.

Landfield, A.W. (1980) 'The Person as Perspectivist, Literalist, and Chaotic Fragmentalist', in A.W. Landfield and L.M. Leitner (eds), *Personal Construct Psychology: Psychotherapy and Personality*, New York: Wiley International.

Lavers, A. (1982) *Roland Barthes: Structuralism and After*, London: Methuen and Co. Ltd.

Leitner, L. (1982) 'Literalism, Perspectivism, Chaotic Fragmentalism and Psychotherapy Techniques', *British Journal of Medical Psychology*, 55: 307–17.

Leman, G. (1970) 'Words and Worlds', in D. Bannister (ed.), *Perspectives in Personal Construct Theory*, London: Academic Press.

Leman-Stefanovic, I. (1987) *The Event of Death: A Phenomenological Enquiry*, Dordrecht: Martinus Nijhoff Publishers.

Leonard, P. (1984) *Personality and Ideology: Towards a Materialist Understanding of the Individual*, London: Macmillan Press.

Lévi-Strauss, C. (1963) *Structural Anthropology*, translated by C. Jacobson and B.G. Schoepf, New York: Basic Books. Originally published 1958 in French.

Lewin, K. (1931) 'The Conflict Between the Aristotelian and Galileian Modes of Thought in Contemporary Psychology', *Journal of General Psychology*, 5: 141–77.

—— (1935) *A Dynamic Theory of Personality*, New York: McGraw-Hill.

Lobkowicz, N. (1967) *Theory and Practice: History of a Concept from Aristotle to Marx*, Notre Dame, Ind.: University of Notre Dame Press.

Lutz, C. (1997) 'Unfenced Constructivisms', *Journal of Constructionist Psychology*, 10, 97–104.

Lyotard, J.F. (1984) *The Postmodern Condition: A Report on Knowledge*, translated by G. Bennington and B. Massumi and with a foreword by F. Jameson, Manchester: Manchester University Press. Original work published 1979 in French.

Mackay, N. (1997) 'Constructivism and the Logic of Explanation', *Journal of Constructivist Psychology*, 10: 339–62.

McMullen, T. (1996) 'John Anderson and Mind as Feeling', *Theory & Psychology*, 6: 153–68.

McWilliams, S.A. (1988), 'On Becoming a Personal Anarchist', in F. Fransella and L. Thomas (eds), *Experimenting With Personal Construct Psychology*, London: Routledge.

—— (1996), 'Accepting the Invitational', in B.M. Walker, J. Costigan, L.L. Viney and B. Warren (eds), *Personal Construct Theory: A Psychology for the Future*, Melbourne: Australian Psychological Society.

Mahoney, M.J. (1988) 'Constructive Matatheory: I. Basic Features and Historical Foundations', *International Journal of Personal Construct Psychology*, 1(1): 1–36.

Mair, M. (1970a) 'The Person in Psychology and Psychotherapy', *British Journal of Medical Psychology*, 43(3): 197–205.

—— (1970b) 'Experimenting with Individuals', *British Journal of Medical Psychology*, 43(3), 245–256.

—— (1985) 'The Long Quest to Know', in F. Epting and A.W. Landfield (eds), *Anticipating Personal Construct Psychology*, Lincoln, Nebr.: University of Nebraska Press.

—— (1989) *Between Psychology and Psychotherapy: A Poetics of Experience*, London: Routledge.

Mancini, F. and Semarari, A. (1988) 'Kelly and Popper: A Constructive View of Knowledge', in F. Fransella and L. Thomas (eds), *Experimenting With Personal Construct Psychology*, London: Routledge.

Mancuso, J.C. (1996) 'Constructionism, Personal Construct Psychology and Narrative Psychology', *Theory & Psychology*, 6: 47–70.

—— (1996) 'The Socializing of Personal Construction', *Theory & Psychology*, 6: 85–92.

Maranell, G.M. (1974) *Responses to Religion: Studies in the Social Psychology of Religious Belief*, Lawrence, Kan.: University of Kansas Press.

Marcuse, H. (1941) 'Some Implications of Modern Technology', *Studies in Philosophy and Social Science*, 9: 414–39.

—— (1968) 'Philosophy and Critical Theory', in *Negations*, Harmondsworth: Penguin. Original essay published 1937.

—— (1969) *Eros and Civilization*, London: Sphere Books Ltd. Original work published 1955.

—— (1970) *One-Dimensional Man*, London: Sphere Books Ltd. Original work published 1964.

—— (1978) 'Interview with Bryan Magee', in B. Magee (ed.) *Men of Ideas: Some Creators of Modern Philosophy*, London: British Broadcasting Corporation.

Margolis, J. (1978) 'Persons and Minds: The Prospects of a Non-reductive Materialism', *Boston Studies in the Philosophy of Science*, 57, Boston: Reidel.

Marshall, J. (1997) 'Michel Foucault: Problematising the Individual and Constituting "the" Self', *Educational Philosophy and Theory*, 29: 32–49.

Marx, K. (1844a) 'The Economic and Philosophical Manuscripts of 1844', in *Collected Works, Vol. 4*, New York: International Publishers.

—— (1844b) 'The Holy Family', in *Collected Works, Vol. 4*, New York: International Publishers.

—— (1845) 'Theses on Feuerbach', in *Collected Works, Vol. 5*, New York: International Publishers.

—— (1845–6) 'The German Ideology', in *Collected Works, Vol. 5*, New York: International Publishers.

Mascolo, M.F. (1994) 'Toward a Social Constructivist Psychology: The Case of Self-evaluating Emotional Development', *Journal of Constructivist Psychology*, 7, 87–106.

Mascolo, M.F. and Dalto, C.A. (1995) 'Self and Modernity on Trial: A Reply to Gergen's "Saturated Self"', *Journal of Constructivist Psychology*, 8: 175–91.

Mascolo, M.F. and Pollack, R.D. (1977) 'Frontiers of Constructivism: Problems and Prospects', *Journal of Constructivist Psychology*, 10(1): 1–6.

Mascolo, M.F., Pollack, R.D. and Fischer, K.W. (1997) 'Keeping the Constructor in Developments: An Epigenetic Systems Approach', *Journal of Constructivist Psychology*, 10: 25–50.

Matthews, M. (1980) 'Knowledge, Action and Power', in R. Mackie (ed.), *Literacy and Revolution: The Pedagogy of Paulo Freire*, London: Pluto Press.

Maturana, H.R. and Varela, F.J. (1980) *Autopoeisis and Cognition: The Realization of the Living*, Boston: Reidel. Original work published 1972.

—— (1987) *The Tree of Knowledge: The Biological Roots of Human Understanding*, Boston: Shambhala. Original work published 1984.

Maze, J.R. (1987), 'John Anderson: Implications of his Philosophical Views for Psychology', *Dialectic* (University of Newcastle, Australia), 30: 50–9.

Mead, G.H. (1948) *Mind, Self and Society*, edited by C.W. Morris, Chicago: University of Chicago Press.

Merleau-Ponty, M. (1962) *Phenomenology of Perception*, translated by C. Smith, London: Routledge. Original work published 1945 in French.

Michael, M. and Kendall, G. (1997) 'Critical Thought, Institutional Contexts, Normative Projects: A Reply to Gergen', *Theory & Psychology*, 7: 37–42.

Mitzman, A. (1969) *The Iron Cage: An Historical Interpretation of Max Weber*, New York: Grosset and Dunlap.

Morris, Van C. (1961) 'Existentialism and the Education of twentieth Century Man', *Educational Theory*, 11: 52–62.

Morrish, I., *Disciplines of Education*, London: George Allen and Unwin Ltd.

Moshman, D. (1982) 'Exogenous, Endogenous, and Dialectical Constructivism', *Developmental Review*, 2(4): 371–84.

Murray, D.L. (1912) *Pragmatism*, London: Constable and Company Ltd.

Neimeyer, R.A. (1985) 'Problems and Prospects in Personal Construct Theory', in D. Bannister (ed.), *Issues and Approaches in Personal Construct Theory*, London: Academic Press.

—— (1988) 'Integrative Directions in Personal Construct Therapy', *International Journal of Personal Construct Psychology*, 1: 283–98.

—— (1995a) 'Limits and Lessons of Constructivism: Some Critical Reflections', *Journal of Constructivist Psychology*, 8: 339–62.

—— (1995b), 'Constructivist Psychotherapies: Features, Foundations, and Future Directions', in R.A. Neimeyer and M.J. Mahoney (eds). *Constructivism and Psychotherapy*, Washington, DC: American Psychological Association.

—— (1997) 'Problems and Prospects in Constructivist Psychology', *Journal of Constructivist Psychology*, 10, 51–74.

Neisser, U. (1967) *Cognitive Psychology*, New York: Appleton-Century-Crofts.

—— (1976) *Cognition and Reality*, London: Routledge and Kegan Paul.

Neu, J. (1977) *Emotion, Thoughts and Therapy*, London: Routledge and Kegan Paul.

Noaparast, K.B. (1995) 'Towards a More Realistic Constructivism', *Advances in Personal Construct Psychology*, 3: 37–59.

Norris, C. (1992) *Uncritical Essays: Postmodernism, Intellectuals and the Gulf War*, London: Lawrence and Wishart.

—— (1993) *The Truth About Postmodernism*, Oxford: Basil Blackwell.

Novak, R.M. (1983) 'Personal Construct Theory and Other Perceptual Pedagogies', in J.R. Adams-Webber and J.C. Mancuso (eds), *Applications of Personal Construct Theory*, New York: Academic Press.

—— (1993), 'Human Constructivism: A Unification of Psychological and Epistemological Phenomena in Meaning Making', *Journal of Constructivist Psychology*, 6: 167–94.

O'Connor, D.J. (1957) *An Introduction to the Philosophy of Education*, London: Routledge.

O'Donohue, W. and Kitchener, R.F. (eds) (1996) *The Philosophy of Psychology*, London: Sage Publications.

O'Farrell, C. (1989) *Foucault: Historian or Philosopher?*, London: Macmillan.

Ogden, C.K. and Richards, I.A. (1972) *The Meaning of Meaning*, tenth edition, London: Routledge and Kegan Paul. Original work published 1923.

O'Hara, M. (1995) 'Is it Time for Clinical Psychology to Deconstruct Constructivism?' *Journal of Constructivist Psychology*, 8, 293–304.

O'Loughlin, M. (1997) 'Corporeal Subjectivities: Merleau-Ponty, Education and the "Postmodern" Subject', *Educational Philosophy and Theory*, 29: 20–31.

O'Neil, W.M. (1987), 'Psychology: Another View', *Dialectic* (University of Newcastle, Australia), 10: 60–2.

Otto, R. (1923) *The Idea of the Holy*, London: Oxford University Press.

Overend, T. (1983) *Social Idealism and the Problem of Objectivity*, St Lucia, Brisbane: University of Queensland Press.

Overend, T. and Lewins, F. (1973). 'A Berger and Luckmann Critique', *La Trobe Sociology Papers, Number 5*, Melbourne: La Trobe University.

Page, C. (1991) 'Philosophical Hermeneutics and Its Meaning for Philosophy', *Philosophy Today*, 35: 127–36.

Pappe, H.O. (1961) 'On Philosophical Anthropology', *Australasian Journal of Philosophy*, 39: 47–64.

Passmore, J. (1973) *Philosophical Reasoning*, London: Duckworth.

—— (1978) *Science and Its Critics*, London: Duckworth.

—— (1985) *Recent Philosophers*, London: Duckworth.

Payne, R. (1967) *The Christian Centuries*, London: W.H. Allen.

Peters, M. and Marshall, J. (1993) 'Beyond the Philosophy of the Subject: Liberalism, Education and the Critique of Individualism', *Educational Philosophy and Theory*, 25: 19–39.

Piaget, J. (1972) *Insights and Illusions of Philosophy*, second edition, translated by W. Mays, London: Routledge. Original work published 1965 in French.

Pocock, D. (1995) 'Searching for a Better Story: Harnessing Modern and Postmodern Positions in Family Therapy', *Journal of Family Therapy*, 17: 149–73.

Polkinghorne, D.E. (1992) 'Postmodern Epistemology of Practice', in S. Kvale (ed.), *Psychology and Postmodernism*, London: Sage Publications.

Pompa, L. (1979) 'Human Nature and the Concept of a Human Science', in G. Tagliacozzo, M. Mooney and D.P. Verene (eds), *Vico and Contemporary Thought*, Atlantic Highlands, NJ: Humanities Press. Original essay published 1976.

Popper, K. (1945) *The Open Society and Its Enemies*, London: Routledge.

—— (1963) *Conjectures and Refutations*, London: Routledge and Kegan Paul.

Popper, K. and Eccles, J.C. (1977) *The Self and Its Brain*, Berlin: Springer International.

Pribram, K.H. (1986) 'The Cognitive Revolution and Mind-brain Issues', *American Psychologist*, 41: 507–20.

Putnam, H. (1987) 'Confrontational Psychology and Interpretation Theory', in R. Born (ed.), *Artificial Intelligence: The Case Against*, New York: St Martin's Press.

Rapp, F. (1982) 'Philosophy of Technology', in G. Floistad (ed.), *Contemporary Philosophy: A New Survey, Vol. 2*, The Hague: Martinus Nijhoff Publishers.

Raskin, J.D. and Epting, F.R. (1993) 'Personal Construct Theory and the Argument Against Mental Illness', *International Journal of Personal Construct Psychology*, 6: 351–70.

Redding, P. (1996) *Hegel's Hermeneutics*, Ithaca, NY: Cornell University Press.

Rhinehart, L. (1971) *The Dice Man*, New York: William Morrow and Co., Inc.

Rickman, H.P. (1976) 'Introduction', in W. Dilthey, *Selected Writings*, Cambridge: Cambridge University Press.

Roazen, P. (1968) *Freud: Political and Social Thought*, New York: Alfred A. Knopf.

Roback, A.A. (1964) *A History of American Psychology*, revised edition, New York: Collier Books.

Robinson, P.A. (1969) *The Freudian Left*, New York: Harper and Row.

Rokeach, M. (1960) *The Open and Closed Mind*, New York: Basic Books.

Rorty, R. (1980) *Philosophy and the Mirror of Nature*, Oxford: Basil Blackwell.

—— (1991) *Objectivity, Realism and Truth*, Cambridge: Cambridge University Press.

Rosen, S. (1991) 'Squaring the Hermeneutic Circle', *Review of Metaphysics*, XLIV(4): 707–28.

Rowe, D. (1978) *The Experience of Depression*, Chichester: John Wiley and Sons.

—— (1982) *The Construction of Life and Death*, Chichester: John Wiley and Sons.

—— (1991) *Wanting Everything*, London: HarperCollins Publishers.

—— (1996) 'The Importance of Personal Construct Psychology', in B.M. Walker, J. Costigan, L.L. Viney and B. Warren (eds), *Personal Construct Theory: A Psychology for the Future*, Melbourne: Australian Psychological Society.

Russell, B. (1954) *The Analysis of Matter*, New York: Dover. Original work published 1927.

—— (1970) *Authority and the Individual*, London: Unwin. Original work published 1949.

—— (1996) 'Why I Am Not a Christian', in J.G. Slater (ed.) *The Collected Papers of Bertrand Russell, Vol. 10*, London: Routledge. Original work published 1927.

Rychlak, J.F. (1970) 'The Human Person in Modern Psychological Science', *British Journal of Medical Psychology*, 43(3): 233–40.

—— (1978) 'Dialectical Features of Kellyian Theorizing', in F. Fransella (ed.), *Personal Construct Psychology 1977*, London: Academic Press.

—— (1985) *A Philosophy of Science for Personality Theory*, second revised edition, Boston: Houghton Mifflin. Original work published 1968.

—— (1988) *The Psychology of Rigorous Humanism*, second edition, New York: New York University Press. Original work published 1977.

—— (1990) 'George Kelly and the Concept of Construction', *International Journal of Personal Construct Psychology*, 3: 7–20.

—— (1991a) *Artificial Intelligence and Human Reason: A Teleological Critique*, New York: Columbia University Press.

—— (1991b) 'The Missing Psychological Links of Artificial Intelligence', *International Journal of Personal Construct Psychology*, 4: 241–9.

—— (1993) 'A Suggested Principle of Complementarity: In Theory not Method', *American Psychologist*, 48: 933–42.

—— (1994) *Logical Learning Theory: A Human Teleology and Its Empirical Support*, Lincoln, Nebr.: University of Nebraska Press.

—— (1996) 'Must Behaviour Be Mechanistic?: Modeling Nonmachines', in W. O'Donohue and R.F. Kitchener (eds), *The Philosophy of Psychology*, London: Sage Publications.

Rychlak, J.F., Barnard, S., Williams, R.N. and Wollman, N. (1989) 'The Recognition and Cognitive Utilization of Oppositionality', *Journal of Psycholinguistic Research*, 18(2): 181–99.

Rychlak, J.F., Stilson, S.R. and Rychlak, L.S. (1993) 'Testing a Predicational Model of Cognition: Cueing Predicate Meanings in Sentences and Word Triplets', *Journal of Psycholinguistic Research*, 22(5): 479–502.

Sadler, J.Z., Wiggins, O.P. and Schwartz, M.A. (eds) (1994) *Philosophical Perspectives on Psychiatric Diagnostic Classification*, Baltimore: Johns Hopkins University Press.

Salmon, P. (1970), 'A Psychology of Personal Growth', in D. Bannister (ed.), *Perspectives in Personal Construct Theory*, London: Academic Press.

Sarbin, T.R. and Mancuso, J.C. (1980) *Schizophrenia: Medical Diagnosis or Moral Verdict*, Elmsford, NY: Pergamon Press.

Sartre, J.P. (1966) *Being and Nothingness*, translated by H.E. Barnes, New York: Philosophical Library. Original work published 1943 in French.

Schalow, F. (1990) 'Is There a "Meaning" of Being?', *Philosophy Today*, 34: 152–62.

Scheer, J.W. (1996) '"Congress" Language, Personal Constructs, and Constructive Internationalism', in B.M. Walker, J. Costigan, L.L. Viney and B. Warren (eds), *Personal Construct Theory: A Psychology for the Future*, Melbourne: Australian Psychological Society.

Scheffler, I. (1965) *Conditions of Knowledge*, Glenview, Ill.: Scott, Foresman.

Schiller, F.C.S. (1926) 'Judgements Versus Propositions', *Mind*, 34: 337–43.

Schleiermacher, F. (1977) *Hermeneutics: The Handwritten Manuscript*, translated by J. Duke and J. Forstman, edited by H. Kimmerle, Atlanta, Ga: The Scholars Press.

Schwab, M. (1989) 'Introduction', in M. Frank, *What is Neostructuralism?*, translated by S. Wilke and R. Gray, Minneapolis: University of Minnesota Press. Original work published 1984 in German.

Scruton, R. (1994) *Modern Philosophy: A Survey*, London: Sinclair-Stevenson.

Searle, J.R. (1995) *The Construction of Social Reality*, New York: Free Press.

Seung, T.K. (1989) 'Kant's Conception of the Categories', *Review of Metaphysics*, 43: 107–32.

Sève, L. (1978) *Man in Marxist Theory and the Psychology of Personality*, translated by J. McGreal, Brighton: Harvester Press. Original work published 1974.

Shearson, W.A. (1975) 'The Common Assumptions of Existential Philosophy', *International Philosophical Quarterly*, 15: 131–47.

—— (1980) *The Notion of Encounter*, Ottawa, Canada: Canadian Association for Publishing in Philosophy.

Shotter, J. (1975) *Images of Man in Psychological Research*, London: Methuen.

—— (1997) 'The Social Construction of Our Inner Selves', *Journal of Constructivist Psychology*, 10: 7–24.

Sigel, I.E. and Holmgren, A. (1983) 'A Constructionist Dialectic View of the Development of the Person: An Update', in J. Mancuso and J. Adams-Webber (eds), *Applications of Personal Construct Theory*, Toronto: Academic Press.

Skinner, B.F. (1971) *Beyond Freedom and Dignity*, New York: Alfred A. Knopf.

Smail, D. (1987) *Taking Care*, London: Dent.

Soffer, J. (1990) 'George Kelly Versus the Existentialists: Theoretical and Therapeutic Implications', *International Journal of Personal Construct Psychology*, 3(4): 357–76.

—— (1993) 'Jean Piaget and George Kelly: Toward a Strong Constructivism', *International Journal of Personal Construct Psychology*, 6: 56–77.

Sokal, A. and Bricmont, J. (1997) *Impostures Intellectuelles*, Paris: O. Jacob.

Solas, J. (1992), 'Ideological Dimensions Implicit in Kelly's Theory of Personal Constructs', *International Journal of Personal Construct Psychology*, 5: 377–92.

—— (1995) 'Grammatology of Social Construing', *Advances in Personal Construct Psychology*, 3: 61–76.

Sorel, G. (1895) 'La Science dans L'Education', *Le Devenir Social* (private translation).

Spinoza, B. (1967) *Ethics*, London: J.M. Dent and Sons Ltd (Everyman Edition). Original work published 1677 in Latin.

Stefan, C. (1977) 'Core Structure Theory and Implications', in D. Bannister (ed.), *New Perspectives in Personal Construct Theory*, London: Academic Press.

Steier, F. (1991a) 'Introduction', in F. Steier (ed.), *Research and Reflexivity*, London: Sage Publications.

—— (1991b) 'Reflexivity and Methodology: An Ecological Constructionism', in F. Steier (ed.), *Research and Reflexivity*, London: Sage Publications.

Stevens, C. (1998) 'A Constructive Alternative: Kelly as a Realist', *Journal of Constructivist Psychology*, 11(4).

Stewart, A.E. and Barry, J.R. (1991) 'Origins of George Kelly's Constructivism in the Work of Korzybski and Moreno', *International Journal of Personal Construct Psychology*, 4: 121–36.

Stirner, M. (1963) *The Ego and His Own: The Case for the Individual Against Authority*, translated by S. Byington, edited by J.J. Martin, New York: Libertarian Book Club. Original work published 1845 in German.

Stojnov, D. (1996) 'Kelly's Theory of Ethics: Hidden, Mislaid, or Misleading?', *Journal of Constructivist Psychology*, 9: 185–200.

Strawson, P.F. (1959) *Individuals: An Essay in Descriptive Metaphysics*, London: Methuen and Co.

Stubenberg, L. (1996) 'The Place of Qualia in the World of Science', in S.R. Hameroff, A.W. Kaszniak and A.C. Scott (eds) *Toward a Science of Consciousness*, Cambridge, Mass.: MIT Press.

Sturrock, J. (ed.) (1979) *Structuralism and Since*, New York: Oxford University Press.

190 *References*

Sturrock, J. (1986) *Structuralism*, London: Paladin (Collins Publishing Group).
Sullivan, E.V. (1984) *A Critical Psychology: Interpretation in the Personal World*, New York: Plenum.
Switzer, D.K. (1970) *Dynamics of Grief: Its Sources, Pain and Healing*, Nashville: Abington Press.
Szasz, T. (1974) *The Myth of Mental Illness: Foundations for a Theory of Personal Conduct*, revised edition, New York: Harper and Row. .
Tagliacozzo, G., Mooney, M. and Verene, D.P. (eds) (1979) *Vico and Contemporary Thought*, Atlantic Highlands, NJ: Humanities Press. Original work published 1976.
Tesconi, C. and Morris, Van Cleve (1972) *The Anti-Man Culture: Bureautechnocracy and the Schools*, Urbana: University of Illinois Press.
Thomas, J. (1984) 'Spinoza as Background to the Ethics of the Frankfurt School', *Dialectic* (University of Newcastle, Australia), 23: 60–6.
Tillich, P. (1952) *The Courage To Be*, New Haven: Yale University Press.
Titchener, E.B. (1928) *A Beginners Psychology*, New York: Macmillan Co.
Todd, N. (1988) 'Religious Belief and PCT', in F. Fransella and L. Thomas (eds), *Experimenting With Personal Construct Psychology*, London: Routledge and Kegan Paul.
Tomkins, S. (1963) 'Left and Right: A Basic Dimension of Ideology and Personality', in R.W. White (ed.), *The Study of Lives*, New York: Atherton Press.
Tönnies, F. (1959) *Community and Society*, translated by C.P. Loomis, New York: Harper and Row. Original work published 1887 in German.
Tucker, D.F.B. (1980) *Marxism and Individualism*, Oxford: Basil Blackwell.
Turkle, S. (1978) *Psychoanalytic Politics*, New York: Basic Books.
Vaihinger, H. (1952) *The Philosophy of the 'As If'*, translated by C.K. Ogden, London: Routledge and Kegan Paul. Original work published 1911 in German.
Van Reijen, W. (1992) 'The Crisis of the Subject: From Baroque to Postmodern', *Philosophy Today*, Winter: 310–23.
Varela, F.J. (1979) *Principles of Biological Autonomy*, New York: Elsevier North Holland.
Vázquez, A.S. (1977) *The Philosophy of Praxis*, translated by M. Gonzalez, London: Merlin Press. Original work published 1966 in Spanish.
Vico, G. (1948) *The New Science*, translated by T.G. Bergin and M.H. Fisch, Ithaca, NY: Cornell University Press. Original work (third edition) published 1744 in Italian.
Voltaire, F.M.A. de (1967) 'Micromagus: A Philosophical Tale', in *Candide and Other Tales*, translated by T. Smollett and revised by J.C. Thornton, introduced by H.N. Brailsford. London: Dent. Original work published 1752 in French.
Walker, B.M. (1990) 'Construing George Kelly's Construing of the Person-in-Relation', *International Journal of Personal Construct Psychology*, 3: 41–50.
—— (1992) 'Values and Kelly's Theory', *International Journal of Personal Construct Psychology*, 5: 259–69.
—— (1996) 'A Psychology for Adventurers: An Introduction to Personal Construct Psychology from a Social Perspective', in D. Kalekin-Fishman and B.M. Walker (eds), *The Construction of Group Realities*, Malabar, Fla: Robert E. Krieger Publishing Company.

Warren, W.G. (1985) 'Personal Construct Psychology and Contemporary Philosophy: An Examination of Alignments', in D. Bannister (ed.), *Issues and Approaches In Personal Construct Theory*, London: Academic Press.

—— (1989) 'Personal Construct Theory and General Trends in Contemporary Philosophy', *International Journal of Personal Construct Psychology*, 2(3): 287–300.

—— (1990a) 'Personal Construct Theory and the Aristotelian and Galileian Modes of Thought', *International Journal of Personal Construct Psychology*, 3(3): 263–80.

—— (1990b) 'Is Personal Construct Psychology A Cognitive Psychology?', *International Journal of Personal Construct Psychology*, 3(4): 393–414.

—— (1991) 'Rising Up From Down Under: A Response to Adams-Webber on Cognitive Psychology and Personal Construct Psychology', *International Journal of Personal Construct Psychology*, 4(1): 43–50.

—— (1992a) 'Personal Construct Theory and Mental Health', *International Journal of Personal Construct Psychology*, 5: 223–38.

—— (1992b) 'Subjecting and Objecting in Personal Construct Psychology', in A. Thomson and P. Cummins (eds), *European Perspectives in Personal Construct Psychology*, Lincoln, Nebr.: European Personal Construct Association.

—— (1993) 'The Problem of Religion for Constructivist Psychology', *Journal of Psychology*, 127: 481–8.

—— (1996) '"The Egalitarian Outlook" as the Underpinning of the Theory of Personal Constructs', in D. Kalekin-Fishman and B.M. Walker (eds), *The Construction of Group Realities*, Malabar, Fla: Robert E. Krieger Publishing Company.

—— (1997) 'Refocussing the Subject: The Anarcho-Psychological Tradition Revisited', *Educational Philosophy and Theory*, 28(1): 89–196.

Waterman, A.S. (1988) 'On the Uses of Psychological Theory and Research in the Process of Ethical Inquiry', *Psychological Bulletin*, 103(3): 283–98.

Weber, M. (1948) *The Protestant Ethic and the Spirit of Capitalism*, translated by T. Parsons, London: George Allen and Unwin. Original work published 1904–5 in German.

Weblin, M.M. (1996) 'The Place of John Anderson in the History of Philosophy', unpublished doctoral thesis, University of New England, Armidale, NSW, Australia.

Williams, R. (1976) *Keywords: A Vocabulary of Culture and Society*, London: Fontana.

Willutzki, V. and Duda, L. (1996) 'The Social Construction of Powerfulness and Powerlessness', in D. Kalekin-Fishman and B.M. Walker (eds), *The Construction of Group Realities*, Malabar, Fla: Robert E. Krieger Publishing Company.

Winter, D.A. (1988) 'Reconstructing an Erection and Elaborating Ejaculation: Personal Construct Theory Perspectives on Sex Therapy', *International Journal of Personal Construct Psychology*, 1: 81–99.

—— (1992) *Personal Construct Psychology in Clinical Practice*, London: Routledge.

Wittgenstein, L. (1953) *Philosophical Investigations*, translated by G.E.M. Anscombe, Oxford: Basil Blackwell.

Woodcock, G. (1986) *The Anarchists*, Harmondsworth: Penguin. Reprinted with postscript.

Wortham, S. (1996) 'Are Constructs Personal?', *Theory & Psychology*, 6: 79–84.

Yorke, M. (1989) 'The Intolerable Wrestle: Words, Numbers, and Meanings', *International Journal of Personal Construct Psychology*, 2: 65–76.

Index

abduction 27
Ackermann, R. 27
Adams-Webber, J. 36, 110, 114, 133
Adler, A. 22
Adorno, T.W. 145
advocacy 50
aesthetics 18
affect 52
agency 95–6
Agnew, J. 4, 131
alienation 11–12, 152
Althusser, L. 147
Amerikaner, M. 119, 143
Anabaptists 153
analytic philosophy 19–20
anarchism 11–12, 138, 153
anarcho-psychologism 2, 14–15, 87
Anderson, J.: influence 62; on being 25;
    on causation 64; on disinterestedness
    85; on ethics 17–18, 34, 63; on Freud
    118; on Hegel 10; on psychological
    science 117; on Vico 42, 43; realist
    position 3, 48–9, 52–6, 71
Anticipation 33
antinomies 46, 48
anxiety 117
Appelbaum, S.A. 23, 169
apperception 46–7
Ardila, R. 111, 128–9, 134
Arendt, H. 161
Aristotle 23, 63, 108, 115, 135–6
Armstrong, D. 17, 48
artificial intelligence 114
Augustine 91
authoritarianism 69, 85, 137–8, 145, 147
authority: alienation 11; individual and
    87; power and 137, 143, 144, 145;
    religion and 152, 153
autopoesis 102

axiology 18

Baker, A.J. 52, 53, 63
Balbi, J. 93, 94
Baldwin, J.M. 24
Bannister, D.: on anxiety 117; on Grid
    Test 131; on personal construct
    psychology 4, 106, 140; on personal
    construct therapy 132; on self
    99–101; on theories 51
Barbu, Z.: on historical psychology 141;
    on individuation 39, 89–90; on
    objectivity 57; on psychology of
    democracy 100, 143, 145–6, 154
Barclay, C.R. 93
Barglow, R. 96
Barry, J.R. 23
Barth, K. 158
Barthes, R. 75
Baum, R.F. 78
Beauvoir, S. de 21, 37
Beethoven, L. van 149
behaviour 109
behaviour therapy 129
behaviourism 105, 129, 141
Being, meaning of 161
belief, religious 152
bereavement 91
Berger, P.L. 61, 62, 64, 67
Bergson, H. 104
Bernstein, R.J. 57, 58, 135, 142, 160
Berzonsky, M.D. 94, 101
Bible 9, 13
Bickhard, M.H. 55, 57, 112, 114, 116
Bios 67, 115
Block, E. 161
Block, N. 105
body 39
Bolton, N. 41, 59, 123–4

Botella, L. 82, 83, 86
Brenkert, G. 62
Brentano, F. 67
Bricmont, J. 74, 86
Bridgman, P.W. 128
Broad, C.D. 18
Brown, P. 132
Brown, S.C. 105
Bubner, R.: on death 91; on Hegel
    studies 12; on Heidegger 159, 165; on
    interconnectedness 49; on
    Kierkegaard 160; on language 161;
    on *phronesis* 162
Buddhism 50
Bugental, E.K. 95
Bugental, J.F.T. 95
Bunge, M. 111, 128–9, 134
Burkitt, I. 66
Burnett, J. 8
Butt, T. 3, 38–9, 71, 102, 169, 172
Button, E. 4, 119

Campbell, N.R. 106, 128
capitalism 9–10, 142
Caponigri, A.R. 43
Caputo, J.D. 161
Carroll, J. 14, 15, 69, 80, 87, 155
categories 16, 35–6
causation 63–4
Chaiklin, S. 82, 120
Chalmers, D.J. 112
change 132
chaotic fragmentalism 118–19
Charlesworth, M. 21, 37
Chiari, G. and Nuzzo, M.L.: on
    biological factors 94; on
    constructivist positions 69–70, 72,
    102, 169; on determinism 117; on
    Kelly 3; on psychotherapy 71, 172; on
    realist constructivism 56
choice corollary 5, 99
Christianity 9–10, 50, 123, 150, 152
Cicero 9
Circumspection–Preemption–Control
    Cycle 33
classification, problem of 3
cognition 52
cognitive: psychology 5, 109–10, 114–15;
    science 3, 105, 109–16, 172
Cohen, A. 74
coherence 56
Colapietro, V.M. 77, 96, 97
commonality corollary 6, 100
community 10, 153

complementarity 67, 69, 172
Comte, A. 24–5
conation 52
conatus 30
Confirmation–Disconfirmation 33
conscientisation 136–7, 140
consciousness: cognitive science 112,
    113; false 146–7; Heidegger on 160;
    Marx on 12; personal construct
    psychology 125; role of language 13
construction corollary 5, 99
constructionism 2–3, 61
constructive alternativism as philosophy
    48–51
Constructive Revision 33
constructivism 2–3, 52, 55, 56; dialectical
    65; ecological 65; endogenous 65;
    epistemological 70, 169; exogenous
    65; hermeneutic 70, 169; in
    psychology 65–71; naive 65–6;
    psychological 70; radical 65–6; social
    65; trivial 65; use of term 61
construing 35
content 33
contrasts 5
convenience, range of 115
cooperation 34
Copernicus 35, 162
correspondence 56
Corsini, R.J. 105
cosmology 17, 21
Cox, L.M. 94, 95, 97
Creativity Cycle 33
Crites, S. 91, 94
critical philosophy 20–1
culture 68
Curtin, T.D. 94
Cushman, P. 95

Dalto, C.A. 82, 86, 97
Dalton, P. 4
Darwin, C. 78
Dascal, M. 74
Davies, P. 17
death 90–1, 160
decision matrices 142
deconstruction 83–4
deduction 27
Deleuze, G. 163
democracy 100, 143, 145–6, 154
democratic mentality 145
dependency 39
Derrida, J. 74, 76, 77, 83, 84, 163
Descartes, R.: dualism 30; epistemology

21, 105, 121; influence on Spinoza 29; on self 89; Vico's criticisms of 42
description 32
determinism 3, 12, 62, 116–18
Deutscher, M. 57
Dewey, J. 25–8; influence 34, 143; Kelly on 23, 28; on philosophy and psychology 48, 49–50, 157; pragmatism 24, 25–8, 56, 71, 83; progressivism 10
dialogue 58, 93, 136, 161
dichotomy corollary 5, 99
difference 15
Dilthey, W.: Holland on 38; method 159; on flow of life 89; on science 109; on time 164; on understanding 159; *verstehen analysis* 106, 126
divisiveness 11
domains 16–19, 23–5
Doniela, B. 32
Dostoevsky, F. 14–15, 80, 87, 88
dread 91
dreams 112–13
DSMs (*Diagnostic and Statistical Manual of Mental Disorders*) 119
dualism 30, 53, 63, 112
Duck, S. 102
Duda, L. 144
Dunnett, G. 4
Durbin, P.T. 129
D'Urso, S. 12

Eccles, J.C. 17
education 10, 12, 47, 142
Edwards, P. 17
egalitarian outlook 145–6, 153
ego 3, 88–9; *see also* self
Ellul, J. 14, 130
emotions 29–30
empiricism 16–17, 25, 27, 34, 53–4, 63
encounter 33, 37, 159
Enlightenment 78, 79, 80, 145
episteme 58
epistemology 16, 23–4, 37, 53, 71, 105
Epting, F.R. 38, 118, 119, 143
Erikson, E.H. 94
Erwin, E. 129
essence 11, 12
ethics 17–18, 21, 31–4, 63, 172
Europe, Kelly in 142
existentialism 15, 37–40; alienation 11; Kelly's relationship with 23, 60; individual 12; Marxism and 88; synthetic philosophy 20

experience corollary 5, 100
Experience Cycle 33
explanation 126, 159, 160

fascism 12, 75
Feuerbach, L.A. 20, 88
Feyerabend, P. 14
fiction 45, 79
Fischer, K.W. 97
Flanagan, O. 112, 113
Floistad, G. 13
Flugel, J.C. 141
flux 49, 89, 161
folk psychology 90
Ford, K.M. 36, 114
Foster, H. 74, 80
Foucault, M.: Frank on 163; on critical ontology 98; on individual 78, 88, 92, 97, 103; on mental illness 118; Scruton on 74; structuralist perspective 75
foundationlessness 83
fragmentalism 118–19
fragmentation 11, 83
fragmentation corollary 5–6, 100
Frank, M. 74, 77, 97–8, 163, 164, 169
Frankena, W. 19
Frankfurt School 13, 14, 20, 32, 62
Frankl, V. 156–7
Fransella, F.: on anxiety 117; on cognitive psychology 110, 114; on Grid Test 131; on Kant's influence 35, 36; on Kelly's religion 150, 152, 172; on personal construct psychology 4, 84, 106, 132, 140; on theories 51
free will 3, 116–18, 156
Freire, P. 13, 136–8, 140
Freud, S.: Anderson on 118; Baum on 78; critique of 133; Frankfurt School perspective 14; ideology 147; influence on Kelly 23, 148; Kelly on 173; on myth 42; psychoanalysis 22; Rat-Man case 75–6
Friedman, M. 97
Fromm, E. 39, 89–90, 141, 145, 157

Gadamer, H.G. 58, 109, 160–1, 162, 163
Galileian mode of thought 108
Galin, D. 113
Gallagher, S. 162
Gallie, W.B. 26
Gardner, H. 110

Geisteswissenschaften 43, 160
Gemeinschaft 10
Georgia, Republic of 142
Gergen, K.J.: on constructivism 61, 65; on folk psychology 90; on postmodernity 81–2, 139; on saturation 94, 95; on self 88, 92; Rychlak on 67, 68
Gestalt psychology 75
Gillett, G. 66, 97, 102
Giorgi, A. 123
Glaserfeld, E. von 65
gnosiology 23–4, 53, 70, 166
Gonçalves, O.F. 94, 97, 103
Gramsci, A. 13
Greeks, ancient 8–9, 22, 73, 110, 145, 152
Greene, M. 125
Grid Test of Schizophrenic Thought Disorder 131
grief 91
guilt 99

Habermas, J.: on human interests 14, 33, 63; on modernity 73; on real world 71; on relativism 161; on self 96
Hameroff, S.R. 111, 112, 113
Hampshire, S. 29
Hardison, O.B. 141
Harré, R. 66, 68, 97, 102
Harriman, P.L. 105
Harris, K. 14
Harris, R. 104
Hawking, S.W. 17, 150–1
Hayes, P.J. 36, 114
Hegel, G.W.F.: dialectic 63; ethics 34; hermeneutics 162–3; historicism 69; influence 10–11, 12, 15, 18, 49, 165, 169; Marxism 20; Mind and Spirit 11, 88; on religion 152–3, 154, 155, 172; phenomenology 6; Spinoza's influence 29; system 22, 73; theory and practice 135–6
hegemony 13
Heidegger, M.: hermeneutics 159–60, 161, 163, 169; on death 90–1; on philosophical anthropology 166; on philosophy 50; on science 14; on technology 130; on time 165; phenomenology 6; realism 60; use of Greek 42, 130, 159
Held, B.S. 56
Henle, M. 131
Heraclitus 6, 8, 49, 89, 104

Herbart, J. 47
hermeneutics 158–64; account of 4; Bernstein on 58; constructive alternativism 50; Kant's work 34; phenomenology 60, 160; radical 161; relationship with personal construct psychology 2, 71, 164–6; relationship with poststructuralism 169
Hess, M. 20
Hillner, K.P. 85, 123, 131
historicism 10
Holland, R.: on existentialism 38; on integrationist perspective 110; on Kelly 23, 38, 41, 138, 142; on personal construct psychology 147–8; on reflexivity 139, 147
Holmgren, A. 66, 101
homo economicus 87–8
Hooker, C.A. 110, 112, 114
Horace 9
Howard, G.S. 56, 94, 95
Huang, Y. 159
Hull, C.L. 68
Hume, D. 18, 29, 65
Hundert, E.M. 56
Husain, M. 33, 36
Husserl, E.: on crisis of rationalism 157; on facts and ideas 2; on origins of philosophy 157; on psychologism 121, 123–4; phenomenology 6, 15, 29, 159; realism 60
hypothesis 27, 45, 134

ICD-10 (*International Classification of Disease*, 10th revision) 119
idealism 12, 52–60, 62–3, 77, 137
ideas, innate 16
identity 94, 104
ideology 88, 141, 146–50
illness 91
individual: anarcho-psychological tradition 14–15; capitalism and 9; constructive alternativism 48; existentialism 12; functioning of 172; Hegel on 34; hermeneutics 164; loss of 81; notion of 3, 87, 145; personal construct psychology 72; stress on 172
individual corollary 5, 99
individuality 87
individuation 39, 89–90
induction 27
inquiry 34, 50, 85
institution 68

instrumentalism 26–7
interpretation 35, 58, 158, 164
Investment 33

Jahoda, M. 110
James, W.: influence 97, 112; influence
  on Kelly 23; neutral monism 25; on
  psychology 120, 123, 128; on self 89,
  100; pragmatism 26, 83
Jennings, J.L. 124–5
Jesus 152–3, 172
John, I.D. 156
Johnson, G.A. 39, 104
Jones, H.G. 72
judgements 121–2
Jung, C.G. 22, 23, 39, 89–90
Jung, M. 26, 159
justice 42
Justinian 9

Kalekin-Fishman, D. 66, 98, 143, 145
Kamenka, E. 64
Kant, I. 34–7; antinomies 46; categories
  16, 35–6, 46; critique of 36, 66;
  hermeneutics 162–3; influence 65, 73,
  124; influence on Kelly 29, 36–7, 60;
  on apperception 46; on means and
  ends 146; questions of philosophy 4,
  15, 22, 167; Tomkins on 149
Kaszniak, A.W. 111, 112, 113
Kelly, G.A.: (1955/1991) 1, 4–5, 23–4, 25,
  27, 28, 35, 38–9, 41, 48, 49, 50, 51, 52,
  56, 59, 70, 74, 86, 102, 110, 111, 115,
  116–17, 125, 128, 131, 132, 133, 134,
  142, 144, 164, 165, 166, 168, 171, 173;
  (1958/1979a) 122; (1958/1979b) 133,
  138; (1961/1979c) 122; (1962/1979d)
  33; (1962/1979e) 118; (1962/1996)
  141–2, 149; (1963) 6; (1963/1979f)
  132, 138; (1963/1979g) 133, 135;
  (1964/1979h) 47, 133, 134;
  (1965/1979i) 131, 132; (1965/1979j)
  120, 127, 152; (1966/1979k) 122, 138,
  139, 168; (1966/1979l) 132; (1970) 33,
  51, 59
Kendall, G. 82
Kendler, H.I. 131
Kierkegaard, S. 91, 160
Kitchener, R.F. 90, 105, 111, 114
knowledge 14, 16–17, 24, 42, 81;
  epistemological question 24;
  evaluative question 24; genetic
  question 24; methodological question

24; pedagogical question 24;
  sociology of 61
Koch, S. 85, 109, 130
Kodis, J. 46
Kolakowski, L. 64, 149
Korzybski, A. 23
Krippendorf, K. 66
Krishna, D. 68
Kropotkin, P. 11, 153
Kuhn, T. 13, 63, 106
Kvale, S. 80–1

labour 11
Lacan, J. 75, 163
Lakatos, I. 14
Landfield, A.W. 118, 143, 150
language 13, 43, 158, 161
latencies 29–31
Lavers, A. 75
Lebenswelt 15, 164
Leibniz, G.W. 46, 89
Leitner, L. 118
Leman, G. 23, 84
Leman-Stefanovic, I. 91
Leonard, P. 12, 62
Lévi-Strauss, C. 75, 76
Lewin, K. 23, 85, 107–8, 131
Lewis, F. 62
Life, meaning of 156, 166
linguistics 13, 23
literalism 118–19
Lobkowicz, N. 135–6
Locke, J. 31, 65, 89
logic 18, 43, 48–9, 121, 123, 169
Logos 67, 115
love 34, 152, 153, 154
Luckmann, T. 61, 62, 64, 67
Luther, M. 9
Lutz, C. 137
Lyddon, W.J. 94, 95, 97
Lyotard, J.F. 78–9, 163

Mackay, N. 52
McMullen, T. 52, 53
McWilliams, S.A. 67–8, 138
Mahoney, M.J. 35, 44, 47, 51, 60
Mair, M.: ethics 32–3; on language 83–4,
  93, 140; on philosophical
  anthropology 167; on psychotherapy
  3, 71; on self 101
Mancini, F. 70
Mancuso, J.C. 66, 101, 119, 120, 133
Maranell, G.M. 151

Marcia, J.E. 94
Marcuse, H.: critics of 154; on
    capitalism 62; on change 68; on
    individual 87; on language 13; on
    science and technology 14, 130;
    philosophical anthropology 167, 168
Margolis, J. 56
Marshall, J. 88
Marx, K.: alienation 11, 152; Baum on
    78; critics of 154–5; determinism 62,
    64; ideology 146, 148; influence 21;
    methodology 76; on individual 12; on
    religion 10, 151; philosophy of
    science 14; *praxis* 136, 139; social
    theory 171; Stirner on 68–9, 88, 103
Marxism: causation 63–4; determinism
    12, 63–4; Frankfurt School 62;
    historical materialism 76; ideology
    147; individual 12, 88; libertarian
    strand 153; philosophy of science 14;
    praxis 136, 139; relationship with
    anarcho-psychological tradition 2;
    relationship with existentialism 88,
    103; relationship with personal
    construct psychology 84
Mascolo, M.F. 82, 86, 97, 102
Matthews, M. 137
Maturana, H.R. 70, 83, 94, 102
Maze, J.R. 52
Mead, G.H. 26, 89, 159
meaning 53, 67, 167
memory 91
mental illness, concept of 3, 118, 126–7
mental representation 110
Merleau-Ponty, M. 38–9, 41, 57, 98, 104
metanarratives 78–9
metaphysics 8, 17, 120
metatheory 51
method 58, 159
methodological essentialism 10
Michael, M. 82
Mill, J.S. 21
mind: Hegel on 11, 88; idealism 17;
    James on 113; Kant on 36; Spinoza
    on 31; *tabula rasa* 16; Vico on 42
minimum realism 56
Mitzman, A. 10, 69
modernity 3, 78–80
modes 19–21
modulation corollary 5, 100
monism 25, 30, 53, 63; neutral 25, 112;
    substantival 25
Mooney, M. 44
morals 17–18, 21, 153

Moreno, J.L. 23
Morris, Van C. 38, 130
Morrish, I. 27
Moshman, D. 65
Murray, D.L. 26
Musgrave, A. 14
Myers, P.R. 94
myth 42, 79, 163, 165

narrative 94, 95, 163
naturalism 54, 157
Naturwissenschaften 43
Neimeyer, R.A. 4, 23, 95–6, 110, 137–8
Neisser, U. 109, 111
neostructuralism 74, 97, 164
Neu, J. 29
New Left 153
Nietzsche, F. 14–15, 65, 68–9, 87
Noaparast, K.B. 55, 57, 71, 169
normative philosophy 19
Norris, C. 79, 86, 161
noumenal world 35
Novak, R.M. 28, 168
Nuzzo, M.L. *see* Chiari

objectivism 157
objectivity 45, 53, 57–9
O'Connor, D.J. 51
O'Donohue, W. 90, 105, 111, 114
O'Farrell, C. 92
Ogden, C.K. 44
O'Hara, M. 134
O'Loughlin, M. 40, 98
O'Neil, W.M. 52
ontology 17, 37, 48, 159–60
operationalism 128
oppositionality 116
organisational corollary 5, 99
Otto, R. 151
Overend, T. 54, 62, 63

Page, C. 161
Pappe, H.O. 167
Passmore, J.: on knowledge 17; on
    language 97; on monism 25; on
    philosophy 74, 78; on philosophy of
    science 13, 106
Payne, R. 9, 152
Peirce, C.S.: decentring of subject 77;
    influence 26, 34, 164; philosophical
    perspective 28; pragmatism 26, 83,
    158; retroduction 27
perception 46

percepts 112
Perry, R.B. 26
person 93–4, 172
personality 12, 71, 107, 165
perspectivism 118–19
Peters, M. 88
phenomenal world 35
phenomenalism 53
phenomenology: Anderson on 52; Heidegger's work 159–60; Husserl's work 15, 60, 124, 159; Jennings' work 124–5; Kelly's rejection of 41; relationship with personal construct psychology 6, 23, 41–2
philosophy: analytic 19–20; constructive alternativism as 48–51; critical 20–1; normative 19; of science 3, 13, 14, 105–9; political 19; social 18–19; speculative 20; synthetic 20
phronesis 58, 162, 169
Physikos 67
Piaget, J. 66, 101, 125
Plato 8–9, 21–2, 69
pluralism 30, 53, 54, 63
Pocock, D. 93
Polanyi, M. 101
political philosophy 19
politics 141–5
Polkinghorne 83, 86
Pollack, R.D. 97
Pompa, L. 44
Popper, K. 10, 13, 17, 69, 70
positivism 24–5, 53, 54, 63
postmodernity: Block on 161; modernity and 78–80; psychology and 80–6, 172; status 3, 74
poststructuralism 73–4, 75–8, 85–6
potential, human 4, 168
power 11, 13, 92–3, 137, 141–5
practice 135, 169
pragmaticism 26
pragmatism: compromise perspective 16–17; Dewey and 24, 25–8; Noaparast's conception 56; personal construct psychology 165; phenomenology and 71, 158; self 96
praxis: Gadamer's approach 58; personal construct psychology 2; personal construct psychotherapy 4, 129, 131, 135–9, 140
predication 116
Preemption Cycle 33
prejudice 124–5
Pribram, K.H. 111

problems 50
progressivism 10
propositions 121
proscription 32, 148
Protagoras 28
Protestantism 9–10, 138
psychoanalysis 62, 75, 141
psychodrama 23
psychologic 167
psychologism 121, 123
psychology 65–71; applied 128, 129, 131–5; clinical 3, 105, 118–20, 128–9, 133–4, 165; cognitive 5, 109–10, 114–15; critical 4; radical 132; use of term 131
psychotechnics 128
psychotechnology 128–30
psychotherapy 3, 71, 131–3, 138, 140, 172
Putnam, H. 111

qualia 112
questioning 165
Quintilian 9

range corollary 5, 100
Rapp, F. 130
Raskin, J.D. 118
Rat-Man case 75–6
rationalism 12, 16–17, 27, 34, 54, 63, 157
realism: Anderson's position 3, 52–5; idealism and 52–60, 63, 70; minimum 56; personal construct psychology 3, 50, 59, 70–1, 173; *praxis* 137
reason 14, 157, 165
Redding, P. 34, 73, 162–3
reflection 107, 160
reflexivity 109, 139, 147, 164
Reformation 145
relativism 17, 53, 55, 58, 63, 76, 82–3
religion 150–4; analytic philosophy 20; Kelly's position 138, 150, 172; philosophical point of view 50; Protestantism 9–10, 138; Roman Catholicism 9, 138
Renaissance 145
Repertory Grid Test 144
retroduction 27
Rhinehart, L. 100
Richards, I.A. 44
Rickman, H.P. 159
Roazen, P. 141
Roback, A.A. 23

Robinson, P.A. 141
Rokeach, M. 145
Roman Catholicism 9, 138
Rorty, R. 28
Rosen, S. 35, 164
Rousseau, J.J. 10, 153–4
Rowe, D.: on personal construct
    psychology 98, 156–7; on power 143,
    144–5; on proof 123; on self 94; on
    significance 84; on Vico 44
Russell, B. 25, 149
Rychlak, J.F.: on concept of
    construction 68; on cognitive science
    110, 111, 114; on Kant 35; on logic
    123; on logical learning theory 115;
    on *Logos* 67; on oppositionality 116;
    on philosophy of science 106–7; on
    self 97; on *Socius* 67; postmodern
    thought 85; principle of
    complementarity 67, 69, 172
Rychlak, L. S. 115, 116

Sadler, J.Z. 119
Salmon, P. 66
Sarbin, T.R. 119, 120
Sartre, J.P. 37, 38–9, 91, 137, 143
saturation 94, 95
Saussure, F. de 75, 76
Scandinavia 142
Schalow, F. 161–2
Scheer, J.W. 142
Scheffler, I. 24
Schiller, F.C.S. 43, 121
Schleiermacher, F. 158–9, 163, 164
Schwab, M. 163–4
Schwartz, M.A. 119
science 13–14, 42–3; cognitive 3, 105,
    109–16, 172; new 44; philosophy of 3,
    13, 14, 105–9; religion and 150, 154
Scott, A.C. 111, 112, 113
Scruton, R. 17, 28, 73–4, 76, 78
Searle, J.R.: external realism 56; Frank
    on 164; postmodernism 86;
    poststructuralism 77; social reality
    67–8, 74, 84
sedimentation 38–9
self: as agent 95, 96; as process 38, 94–5;
    constructing selves 93–8; decentred
    and recentred subjects 92–3; in
    personal construct psychology
    99–103, 171; notion of 3, 39–40,
    87–92; transcendent 95
self-acquaintance 97
self-reflection 107

self-understanding 97
selves, constructing 93–8
Semarari, A. 70
sense impressions 16
Seung, T.K. 36
Sève, L. 12, 62
sex therapy 132
Shearson, W.A. 11, 21, 37
Shotter, J. 32–3, 90, 95, 96–7, 172
Sigel, I.E. 66, 101
signifier 75
Sittlichkeit 34, 153
Skinner, B.F. 141
Smail, D. 144
Smith, T.S. 93
social action 102, 169
social constructionism 1–2, 55, 62–6,
    148, 171–2
social philosophy 18–19
social-political 141–5
social theory 61–4
sociality 42, 153
sociality corollary 6, 100
society 68
sociology of knowledge 61
Socius 67
Socrates 8–9
Soffer, J. 40, 66
Sokal, A. 74, 86
Solas, J. 83, 84, 147, 148
Sophists 8–9
Sorel, G. 85
soul 17
Soviet Union 142
Soyland, A.J. 156
speculative philosophy 20
Spinoza, B. 29–31; influence 6, 22, 60,
    154; interconnected reality 49; on self
    89
Spirit 11, 17, 88
Stefan, C. 139, 147
Steier, F. 65
Stevens, C. 56, 71
Stewart, A.E. 23
Stilson, S.R. 115, 116
Stirner, M. 14–15, 68–9, 87, 88, 103, 109
Stojnov, D. 32–3, 34
Strawson, P.F. 89
structuralism 73–4, 75–8, 163, 164
Stubenberg, L. 112
Sturrock, J. 75, 77
subjectivity 57–9, 94, 113, 145, 172
subjects, centred and decentred 92–3
submission 88

Sullivan, E.V. 4, 85
Switzer, D.K. 91
synthetic philosophy 20
Szasz, T. 118

tabula rasa 16
Tagliacozzo, G. 44
techne 58, 130, 131
technology 14, 128–30
telosponse 115–16
Tesconi, C. 130
Thales 8
theory: meaning of term 50–1, 135;
    types of 32
thinking 51, 130
Thomas, J. 32
thought 45
Tillich, P. 151
time 164–5
Titchener, E. 128
Todd, N. 151
Tomkins, S. 149
Tönnies, F. 10
totality 49
truth: religion and 152; theory of 26
Tucker, D.F.B. 62
Tucson Conference (1994) 112
Turkle, S. 75–6

understanding 126, 159, 160–1
United States, conceptions of 142
utility 14

Vaihinger, H. 44–8; disability 44–5, 69;

influence 29, 60, 79, 134; on Kant 37,
    46
values 18, 107
Van Reijen, W. 88
Varella, F.J. 70, 83, 94, 102, 117
Vázquez, A.S. 136
Verene, D.P. 44
verstehen analysis 106, 126
Vico, G. 29, 42–4, 60, 79, 106, 109
Voltaire 20

Walker, B.M.: on Kelly 32, 148; on self
    98, 101, 104; on social
    constructionism 66, 144, 145
Warren, W.G.: (1985) 23, 25, 41, 44, 52,
    55, 71, 84, 103; (1989) 41; (1990a)
    106, 107; (1990b) 29, 110, 114; (1991)
    110, 114; (1992a) 143; (1992b) 93;
    (1993) 150, 152; (1994) 57; (1996)
    143, 145; (1997) 96
Waterman, A.S. 31, 33
Weber, M. 10, 45, 69
Weblin, M.M. 53
Whitehead, A.N. 149
Wiggins, O.P. 119
Williams, R. 68, 146
Willutzki, V. 144
Winter, D.A. 4, 132
Wittgenstein, L. 20, 120–1, 129
Woodcock, G. 153
Wortham, S. 66

Yorke, M. 43

Zeno 18